PRAISE FOR *THE MINISTRY OF THIN*

'A very honest, intelligent reflection on the causes and effects of society's obsession with thin.'
Dr Linda Papadopoulos

'The Ministry of Thin *is frank, funny, and fascinating – I wanted to shout "hear, hear" at the end of almost every sentence.'*
Anne H. Putnam, author of *Navel Gazing: One Woman's Quest for a Size Normal*

PRAISE FOR *AN APPLE A DAY*

'Frank and compelling... made me understand anorexia in a way I never have before.'
Woman's Hour, BBC Radio 4

'The contrast between her privileged life and her personal misery is strikingly established in this book before she begins to deal positively with her long-standing 'addiction to hunger'...
'Coming out' about her condition and narrating the process of recovery has been as much agony as therapy, but it has been a needful exercise for the writer and her support group of readers.'
The Times

'Emma is highly intelligent and self-aware, and she is courageously willing in her memoir to depict the least attractive aspects of anorexia – the intense self-absorption, and troubling mixture of secrecy and attention-seeking... this is a candid, generous and readable account of a very intractable condition.'
Mail Online

'*It takes guts to admit something's wrong and to resolve to do something about it. It takes even more to do your therapy in public... it's clear that Emma Woolf's column 'An Apple a Day' about her recovery from anorexia has helped many by articulating some complex truths about anorexia, and charting a way forward into recovery.*'
MIND, Nomination for Journalist of the Year 2012

'*In* An Apple a Day *Emma comes across as brave, real and determined. I'm sure that in sharing her story many others will be encouraged to speak out from the stigma of this horrible illness and realise that there is a life worth living beyond calorie counts and scales. It is a battle worth fighting.*'
Grace Bowman, author of *Thin*

'An Apple a Day *tells a powerful story, heart-warming and heart-rending by turns. It is ultimately a story filled with hope, and Emma Woolf's moving, deeply personal account of her journey out of anorexia will bring that hope to so many more people trapped by this dreadful illness.*'
Susan Ringwood, Chief Executive, Beat

'*An insightful and fascinating read for everyone, whether they've been touched by eating disorders or not.*'
Booklist (USA)

'*Her perceptive and articulate account is frank about the mental torment she endured without being morose. Insightful and informative, with fresh insights into the nature of eating disorders.*'
Kirkus Reviews (USA)

'Eloquent, profoundly moving, romantic, and, at times, shocking candid, Emma's fearless and honest account is ultimately one of hope.'
Spirit FM Book Club

'a powerful and heartfelt read... If you read one thing this year, make it An Apple a Day.'
PopGoesCulture2013.wordpress.com

TWEETS

'Finished the most wonderful & inspirational book I've read in ages. Thank u @EJWoolf I look forward to your next #anappleaday'

'@EJWoolf thank you for your beautiful &inspiring book. It makes me believe that after 8 years of hell, I can make it through and really live'

'An unflinching exposé of our obsession with thin'
@VWYoga (Victoria Woodhall, YOU Magazine)

'When you read a book and you feel like someone has poked around in your head and put the thoughts on paper. @EJWoolf's book is like that'

EMAILS FROM READERS

'*If I hadn't read* An Apple a Day, *then I am not sure I would be here today.*'
Hannah

'*I want to thank you for sharing your story: I am sure that I am not alone in feeling that you somehow put pen to paper and convey the exact thoughts storming around in my head that I myself could not rationalise, much less make coherent. Emma: you are doing a fantastic job.*'
Beth

'*Thank you for sharing your story, for writing this book... Page after page, words after words I've seen myself printed on a book and had an overwhelming feeling of gratitude.*'
Nick

'*When I say* Apple *was inspiring, I really do mean it... This has been a massive, massive help to kickstarting my road to recovery.*'
Imogen

'*I cried and I laughed, and at every page found myself wanting to earmark it and use your very words to express what I have felt on so many occasions, and what I still now feel every day in some way.*'
Catriona

To Cecil and Jean Woolf

THE MINISTRY OF THIN

Summersdale Publishers Ltd
46 West Street
Chichester
West Sussex
PO19 1RP
UK

www.summersdale.com

Printed and bound by CPI Group (UK) Ltd, Croydon, CR0 4YY

ISBN: 978-1-84953-412-3

Substantial discounts on bulk quantities of Summersdale books are available to corporations, professional associations and other organisations. For details contact Nicky Douglas by telephone: +44 (0) 1243 756902, fax: +44 (0) 1243 786300 or email: nicky@summersdale.com.

THE
MINISTRY
OF THIN

*How the pursuit
of perfection got
out of control*

EMMA WOOLF

summersdale

ABOUT THE AUTHOR

Emma Woolf is the great-niece of Virginia Woolf. After studying English at Oxford University she worked in publishing, before becoming a full-time writer. She is a columnist for *The Times* and also writes for *The Independent*, *The Mail on Sunday*, *Harper's Bazaar*, *Red*, *Grazia* and *Psychologies*. She was a co-presenter on Channel 4's *Supersize vs Superskinny*; other media appearances include *Newsnight*, *Woman's Hour* and *Radio 4's Four Thought*.

Emma's first book, *An Apple a Day: A Memoir of Love and Recovery from Anorexia* was published in 2012 and shortlisted for the Beat Award for Recovery Inspiration. She was also nominated for Mind's Journalist of the Year. She lives in London. You can follow Emma on Twitter: @ejwoolf.

CONTENTS

INTRODUCTION

Welcome to the Ministry of Thin. All members are welcome and there's no charge – in fact you're signed up automatically at birth. Obviously every organisation needs rules and regulations – these are simple, effective and will last a lifetime:

1. If you aren't thin you aren't attractive.
2. Being thin is more important than being healthy.
3. You must buy clothes, cut your hair, starve yourself, do anything to look thinner.
4. You will not eat without feeling guilty.
5. You will not eat fattening food without punishing yourself afterwards.
6. You will count calories and restrict intake accordingly.
7. What the scale says is the most important thing.
8. Losing weight is good; gaining weight is bad.
9. You can never be too thin.
10. Being thin and not eating are signs of true willpower and success.

The 'thin commandments' (from eatingdisordersonline.com), originally intended to illustrate how extreme some weight-loss behaviour can become, have been taken up as 'thinspiration' mantras on pro-anorexia and pro-bulimia websites. It's easy to dismiss these commandments as dangerous, sick, disordered... but take another look. These have become the *female* commandments, whose basic principles now govern many of our lives. The chances are, if you're female, you'll identify with some of these rules, even if you don't follow them all.

Of course there are still women out there who eat, dress and express themselves with absolute confidence, who mean it when they say they love their bodies and never think about their weight – and that's a wonderful thing. There are cultures in which the rounder female form is preferred to the slender, and developing countries in which food itself is scarce, which don't have the luxury of dieting or body anxiety. But countless surveys have shown that the vast majority of us in the developed Western world would like to be thinner. We worry about our weight constantly, and we believe our lives would be better if we could shift the extra pounds, kilos or stones. Women routinely place losing weight above work goals, health or relationships; a US study in 2011 reported that one in six women would choose to be blind rather than obese, others would prefer herpes or alcoholism to being overweight.

And it's not just women who suffer from negative body image. In 2012 BBC News reported a survey from the Centre for Appearance Research at the University of the West of England in which 4 out of 5 male respondents said they were 'unhappy' with their weight. Among the men (with an average age of forty), the main body issues were 'beer bellies' and lack of muscles – with 60 per cent saying that their arms, chests and stomachs were not muscular enough. Thirty-five per cent of the men even said they would exchange a year of their life to achieve their ideal body weight or shape.

It doesn't need to be this extreme: the chances are, if you're a woman in the twenty-first century reading this, you will have felt some of the pressures and identify with some of the anxieties I explore in this book. As women, our perspectives will vary, from those who would simply like to be more toned and a few pounds lighter, to those who avoid looking at themselves in the mirror or never walk around in front of their partner naked, or those who actively hate their bodies, or deny themselves food when hungry, eat or starve in secret, or those who simply don't feel good about the way they look.

But what is the Ministry of Thin? Perhaps you don't want to be a member, perhaps you don't remember signing up for it. And that's the point. The majority of us, sane, independent, confident women like you and me, don't want to be part of it. We're well aware of the paradox of being caught up in the collective female pursuit of thin while seeing it for what it is.

And we *are* independent, in so many ways – fearless, feminist, sometimes fierce in standing up for ourselves and others. We're in charge of our careers, our fertility, our money; we own property, we use our voting rights, we bring up our families with or without men.

Of course there remain serious gender inequalities: the earnings gap between men and women is still around 13 per cent in the public sector, and around 20 per cent in the private sector. Women in high-flying jobs earn almost half a million pounds less over the course of their working lives than men with identical careers, according to the Chartered Management Institute (November 2012). Women are less likely to receive a bonus and more likely to be made redundant.

Although the number of senior women in FTSE 100 companies is rising, they still make up barely 17 per cent and there are currently only three female FTSE 100 Chief Executives. Ambitious men are considered successful; ambitious women are considered a bit, well, pushy. When is the last time you heard a man called 'bossy'? Industry studies show that UK companies are spectacularly unsuccessful at promoting women, and that women are routinely penalised for requesting maternity leave or for taking career breaks to bring up children. For all the promise of flexible working, the so-called 'motherhood penalty' is alive and well in UK workplaces.

More than forty years after the Equal Pay Act was passed, pay between women and men is still not equal. Depressingly, the only professions in which women can realistically expect to earn more than men are prostitution, modelling and pornography. Female entrepreneurs also do well when pay is determined on actual business performance and growth, rather than decided by male bosses. A global survey has found that self-made women earn on average 17 per cent more than men (Barclays Wealth & Asset Management, January 2013).

The organisation Women in Journalism recently reported that 83 per cent of contributors and presenters on Radio 4's *Today* programme are, guess what, male. Seventy-eight per cent of front-page bylines in national newspapers are male, and the majority of experts quoted are male; women most often appear in newsprint as victims, sex symbols or married to famous men. To illustrate this point, the three most photographed females of recent years are: the Duchess of Cambridge; her sister Pippa Middleton; and Madeleine McCann, the little girl who disappeared in Portugal in 2007. When the girlfriend of Paralympic athlete Oscar Pistorius was shot dead on Valentine's Day 2013, she fulfilled all these criteria: Reeva Steenkamp was not only a glamour model, she was also the girlfriend of a famous man, and a victim. Photographs of the dead woman in a bikini appeared on the front page of many tabloid newspapers while she was still in the mortuary.

The Church of England's General Synod voted in late 2012 against the ordination of women bishops. Interestingly, it was the laity, not the clergy, who narrowly tipped the balance in this vote, but the end result is the same. As many commentators pointed out, women do the majority of work and ministry within the church, but they are still unable to take up their rightful places. It may be the twenty-first century, but the failed attempt to shatter this 'stained-glass ceiling' is a reminder of the old-fashioned sexism which remains entrenched in many of our national institutions.

Despite all this, women are not weak or powerless. We run successful businesses and govern countries; we write books and direct films; we win Olympic medals and Nobel Prizes. Just the other day my boyfriend said: 'Basically, women are better than men at everything.' He sounded surprised, as if this had only just occurred to him. It's not a level playing field for us, there are many glaring inequalities, but we achieve all that men achieve and more.

And yet... There is still a consensus on what women should look like; a near-universal acknowledgement that a thinner body is a superior body. How can we be so strong and yet so idiotic? What is the desire to lose weight really about? Why do we allow the thin-rules to brainwash us?

*

Maybe we were recruited into the Ministry of Thin the day we were born female, or the day we were first dressed in pink, or realised we shouldn't play in the mud with our brothers because pretty girls stay clean. Maybe it was when we first glanced in the mirror and felt rounded, or tubby, or wrong – more than half of three- to six-year-old girls say they feel 'fat'. Or maybe it was the day we first picked up a razor aged eleven or thirteen or fifteen and began the lifelong mowing of body hair.

You may well say that you prefer to look this way – the way women are supposed to look – hairless and smooth, your skin tanned, your eyebrows neatly groomed. And I do too. But is it really a preference: is it OK to say no? When you consider the outcry following the appearance of Julia Roberts on the red carpet *with unshaven armpits* (years ago now, and still notorious) it's debatable whether choice exists any longer.

I'm not demanding that we all stop 'maintaining' ourselves – grow our body hair, throw away our cosmetics, stop exercising. Just that it shouldn't be such a massive deal when we choose not to. As women, our appearance should be a matter of preference, the way a man chooses whether to grow a beard, or not to bother about his receding hairline. We should be able to make up our minds, and I don't believe we do. It's not a choice when there is no choice at all.

The simplest thing, of course, would be to fight back. To stand up to the depilation dictators, to ignore all diet and detox regimes, to embrace ageing, wrinkles and grey hair. It's easier said than done. There are plenty of women who don't wear make-up or dye their hair (although going grey is often seen as 'brave') but the weight issue touches almost everyone. People, especially women, are judged on their bodies. And food, far from being a source of energy and enjoyment, has become a battleground of guilt and shame and excess and starvation. Everywhere we look, success and sexiness and happiness seem to belong to the thin.

In essence, the Ministry of Thin operates from within us, consciously or not, an internal policeman which tells us that thinner is better. To revolt, you need something to revolt against, and the Ministry of Thin isn't that clear-cut. It's the rules, pressures and expectations we live with, it's the media, it's men and it's other women. Hardest of all to stand up to, it's the mirror – it's ourselves.

We first absorb the thin rules as young girls from our mothers, sisters and friends. In adolescence they are reinforced by magazines, boyfriends, and the world around us. By adulthood, wanting to be thinner is just another one of the curious non-essential and yet essential rules to which women adhere: just as we remove our body hair and wear make-up, we worry about our weight, we despair of our bodies, we try not to eat too much, we force ourselves to go to the gym, we feel fat, we diet. There is absolutely nothing unusual about these actions or experiences – disliking one's body and wanting to be thinner is the new normal.

Pick up any woman's magazine these days: *Two weeks to your best-ever bikini body; How to lose weight without feeling hungry; Celebs share their diet secrets.* Or listen to any conversation between teenage girls or adult women. A friend recently told me that her seven-year-old daughter's classmates were compiling a list rating each other as 'skinny, medium or fat'. From childhood we know the rules: fat is bad, thin is good. Think of the terms we use to describe our body parts, that ever-expanding litany of hate: cankles, bingo wings, muffin tops, thunder thighs.

Just as sad as the revulsion we mentally direct at our own bodies every day is the outrage we express towards anyone who doesn't feel it. The Ministry of Thin dictates that women should dislike themselves, or at least express proper insecurities, and we feel suspicious of anyone who doesn't. It is a weird inversion of recent feminist advances: in the second half of the twentieth century we began to find our voices, to accept our bodies, to express our sexuality, to be freer in our clothes and movements and actions. This was followed by Millennial post-feminism, where we learned to embrace our femininity, to bake cupcakes in our Cath Kidston pinnies while mastering Cosmo's sex tip of the month, and trying to convince ourselves we were 'having it all'.

Now, whether we're porn-star-waxed and Botoxed to the frozen eyebrows or not, we seem to have settled into quiet despair. For many of us, the energy, the confidence, is gone. Even if you are happy with the way you look, it's probably safer to pretend you're not, or at least to keep quiet about your peculiar ideas. These days we feel obliged to conform to the rule of personal body hatred.

But I refuse to believe that we're just stupid. I don't think we chose to make our lives so difficult; nor that we want to spend our lives feeling hungry, fat, ugly or old. Is this all a huge conspiracy against women? Well, perhaps not, but there are serious commercial players at work here, industries which make billions from convincing us, from an early age, that we need to overhaul our appearance, lose several stone, wax off every trace of body hair, consume only organic or diet foods, hide our flaws with expensive make-up, remodel and improve with surgery – spend more, more, more because we're inadequate as we are. The female body is a commodity, a consumer item; we've become perfectible – and if we don't make constant efforts to modify it, we're letting ourselves go.

These vested interests include the cosmetic and pharmaceutical industries, health and fitness companies, fashion designers, food producers and advertisers, women's magazines, the personal trainers and gym owners and diet gurus and cosmetic surgeons all with something to peddle. Intentionally or not, these massive corporations have created a febrile climate in which it's normal, nay expected, for women to hate their bodies. Labiaplasty (where women undergo painful surgery in order to achieve a 'designer vagina') is on the increase, a Western form of female genital mutilation.

Of course there are countless unspoken rules to being acceptable as a woman – thou shalt not age; thou shalt not be ugly; thou shalt not be too emotionally open, nor too obviously clever – but being thin trumps them all. Wanting to lose weight is the way women identify with each other – complete strangers will bond over a buffet table with the simple phrase: 'I shouldn't, but this just looks too delicious.' Self-deprecating comments about our appearance are a shortcut to female friendship: I recently caught another woman's eye as we both tried on jeans in the changing room at Zara. As we grimaced at our reflections she said: 'I knew I shouldn't have eaten that ice cream last night!'

Wanting to get thin is also the way we keep our own potential selves in check: 'when I lose ten pounds…' It's our excuse for failure in relationships or at work; it's that mythical dress which is two sizes too small which we'll wear when we reach our goal weight.

As someone who has reached that goal weight, dropped those ten pounds (and much, much more) I can tell you that getting thin doesn't solve anything. But the fact remains: losing weight has become for many of us the female holy grail.

*

So what qualifies me to write about our new obsession with skinny? Well, I'm a thirty-something woman, I have sisters in their twenties and forties, female friends across the age range from teenage to menopausal to eighty-something. As a journalist I write about issues that concern women in newspapers and magazines, including dieting, weight and body image.

More importantly, I've been through more than ten years of anorexia. I'm only now properly out the other side. For me, women's attitudes to eating, hunger and their bodies are fascinating and confusing in equal measure. I find myself simultaneously involved and alienated, both a participant and an outsider. Of course I understand what women mean when they talk about food and weight; when they refer to being good (dieting), or feeling guilty (greedy), or treating themselves (cake). I get it when women talk about disliking specific parts of their bodies. But it's hard too, emerging from a decade of severe food restriction, to look around me for examples of how to eat normally, and how to love and live with and accept myself, only to find that the majority of women are struggling with these issues too. Rationally, we must know that getting thinner won't necessarily make us happier or more fulfilled – and yet we never give up trying, or at least thinking that we *should* be trying.

For so long I thought that anorexia was different. For so long I wondered how most women can diet and exercise and not develop a full-blown eating disorder, whereas I started losing weight and exercising excessively and got sucked into the spiral of anorexia. When I see the girls in the office tucking into chocolate brownies for someone's birthday, moments after announcing their new diet regime, I wonder if eating disorders and disordered eating are actually part of the same spectrum; whether self-starvation is simply a more extreme form of female dieting. I see a lot of anxiety about weight around me; I hear a lot of guilt about food. Sometimes it seems that 'normal' dieting and anorexia are worlds apart, sometimes they seem very close.

Over the past two years I've had a weekly column in *The Times*, charting the ups and downs in my personal journey. In 2012 I wrote *An Apple a Day: A Memoir of Love and Recovery from Anorexia*. I should clarify: I don't think my experiences make me special. In fact, part of the joy of *An Apple a Day* has been the realisation that I'm not that different at all. So many 'normal' readers (both male and female) have contacted me to say, I feel this way too. Most of them do not have an actual eating disorder; they simply recognise that they have disordered eating patterns, feel guilty about their hunger, unhappy with their bodies or out of control around food.

In writing about anorexia I have paid a high personal cost (as anyone who chooses to write 'confessionally' will know) and I'm frequently accused of narcissism. But then I remember what Doris Lessing wrote in *The Golden Notebook*, that 'writing about oneself, one is writing about others'. And that has proved to be true.

So, does this make me an expert or a hypocrite? Recovery from anorexia is probably never completely 'over'; I'm aware that it's something I will work at for the rest of my life. There have been setbacks along the way, but the momentum has always been forward. Physically, I am 'recovered': I eat well and have a healthy BMI. After many years of fear, finally I can enjoy food again: breakfast in bed, an anniversary dinner, a picnic in the park. But I remember how it used to be – every Friday before work I would go to see my psychiatrist and he would ask me to step on the scales. I didn't know whether I wanted to see the numbers go up – which would mean that I was winning the fight against anorexia – or go down – which would mean that I was successful as a woman because I was losing weight.

I will try not to refer to my own anorexia too much. But here's what I'd like to understand: if being thin is the answer, what's the question?

*

You may think that writing about this is the worst thing for me to do. But our obsession with skinny is there: it's a fact. In Elizabeth Gilbert's book on marriage, *Committed*, she explores her ambivalence towards the institution of marriage (shortly before she herself is about to marry). At one point she writes: 'The best way I know how to get really granular and intimate with a subject is to write a book about it.'

And that's what I want to do here. My starting point is not that all diets are bad, nor that all body-dissatisfaction is misplaced.

My aim is not to dissuade anyone from losing weight if they need to. I've never blamed the media or others for my eating disorder and I try not to make sweeping generalisations about the 'modern world'. I'm no sociologist, and I will try to steer clear of shouty accusations about the sexist, ageist, patriarchal society which is keeping women down. (Although it's true that hungry women are much less trouble than strong ones, isn't it?)

The twenty-first century must be one of the best and worst times to be a woman: the pressures on us are immense, the opportunities open to us are incredible. But trust me, it's really hard to function when you don't have enough fuel in the tank.

Having recently rejoined the so-called 'normal' world, I'm fascinated by our seemingly obsessive body-narrative; the daily comments we make about ourselves and others – 'You look amazing, have you lost weight?'; 'OMG those jeans are so slimming!'; 'If you see me going near a carb today, shoot me!' I want to examine the automatic negativity we direct towards our bodies almost without registering it: do we want or need to feel this way? Do we consciously allow these thoughts, or are we simply victims? Now that being thin is synonymous with beauty and success, now that losing weight is the goal which most women have in common, I want to get 'granular' with this aspect of being female.

How did we get to a situation where it's normal to be at war with your own body, appetite and needs? Why do we dislike the skin we're in? It's an issue which is wonderfully easy to satirise, but in truth it goes much deeper than 'does my bum look big in this?'

This is about more than just anxious women squeezing themselves into painfully tight Spanx Pants, or teenage girls wanting to look like supermodels, or PMT-driven chocolate-binges, or anorexics starving themselves to death. This is about the worship of the slender figure by women of all ages and walks of life and the widespread depression and despair which results. This is about the dangerous extremes to which women will go to lose weight (yes, that liquid-only Drip Diet) only to gain it all back again and more.

You know that saying: *inside every fat woman there's a thin woman struggling to get out.* It's supposed to be funny, but it's actually quite sad. Think of the psychological damage; the sadness of feeling let down by your own appearance, inwardly thin and outwardly fat, thwarted by your lack of self-control, sabotaged by your greed and fleshiness, so ashamed that you eat in secret, or binge and then purge, or pretend you're not hungry when you are. Look at the tyranny of the diet industry, the impossible size zero culture and the celebrity-obsessed media, the disconnect between the way we ought to look and the way we are. Isn't it time we took this seriously, when the majority of us are living with constant hunger, wasting hours at the gym, detesting our bodies every morning, feeling guilty with every mouthful, putting our lives on hold until we've lost those hateful ten pounds?

Imagine not caring about your so-called flaws or comparing your shape to that of others, imagine never getting depressed by perfect women in advertisements or on television. Imagine eating in response to your hunger cues and not to your emotions, imagine never going on a diet, never using food as a reward or a punishment. Imagine never weighing yourself or even wanting to lose weight. Imagine not having forbidden foods, not ordering a salad when you really want fish and chips, imagine not minding what your friends eat or what size they are.

Some women achieve this enviable equilibrium, but very few. There's probably no such thing as total body confidence; no simple way to operate in our hyper-visual, highly-connected world without the odd wobble. But the modern obsession with losing weight, the fallacy that thinner automatically equals happier, is making many women (and men) unhappy on a daily basis.

According to Montaigne, 'The greatest thing in the world is to know how to belong to oneself.' Not an easy goal, perhaps, but one worth pursuing. There's a real freedom in deciding not to worry about what others think, or say, or look like, or eat. Maybe, by regaining control of our own thoughts and feelings, we can start to belong to ourselves once more.

Chapter 1

THE MINISTRY OF FOOD

Alice and I are walking down the aisle marked Dairy. I take four small tubs of Greek 0% Total yogurt, a couple of raspberry-flavour Muller Lights. I add a four-pack of vanilla probiotic Activias, then a 2-pint carton of skimmed milk. My sister grimaces at the red-top milk – 'Skimmed? That stuff looks like dirty water.' I nod cheerfully, 'I know, tastes like it too.' We turn the corner into the aisle marked Meat, where it's Al's turn to stock up: bacon, chicken and some kind of fish.

At the checkout queue, we look at our baskets: butter, bacon and eggs in hers, muesli, pitta bread, Greek yogurt in mine. I also have apples, broccoli, bananas; Al has sparkling water, salmon, avocado.

See what she's doing; see what I'm doing? Without even thinking about it, we both have our forbidden foods – or if not entirely forbidden, substances we steer clear of. Al never buys coffee or wine, although she will have the occasional cappuccino or glass of wine when she's out. I literally don't go near butter, and I wouldn't know how to cook any of the meat she buys. Odder than her wariness of caffeine, and my strict vegetarianism, is our avoidance of whole food groups. I don't 'do' fat, she doesn't 'do' carbs. A few decades ago these might have seemed strange rules to follow, but these days they're pretty normal. In the twenty-first century most women police their diets in some way.

At the heart of it all is food, or rather our relationship with food. If we just ate to satisfy our hunger, we could have our meat-and-two-veg and leave it there. If calories were simply fuel, we'd consume what our bodies required, and there would be no weight problems. But few of us are that straightforward: we eat in response to emotional cues, not just hunger, we use food as a reward or withhold it as punishment, we bury sadness or despair in eating, we celebrate or console with meals, we demonstrate love and care and nurture through feeding others.

I suppose anorexia has made me hyper-aware of our ever-present food culture. Not that the food is tempting per se – not-eating is the most basic rule you master in anorexia – simply that the enemy is everywhere. Social situations involving food are hard to avoid, and those mantras of my anorexic decade: 'Honestly, I'm not hungry' and 'I'm fine, I just ate' resound in my head.

When I was writing *An Apple a Day*, one of the promises I made was that I would try to be less fearful of fat: 'I will remember that Brazil nuts, olive oil and other essential fats give you shiny hair and great skin, not a fat bum.' I've had some success with this – linseeds and pumpkins seeds for fat, hummus for protein – but I have to be careful. I try to ignore articles in magazines on sinful foods and miracle diets. And when other women are discussing what to eat and what to avoid, I do my best not to take it too seriously.

Bananas, for example. Yesterday a colleague at work commented, 'If I ate bananas I'd have to run about 20 miles a day to burn them off.' It was an offhand comment, said through a mouthful of chocolate brownie, and I shouldn't even have given it head-space. But bananas used to be problematic for me – they have a reputation for being higher in calories than other fruits, full of carbs. I felt a residual twinge of anxiety because I eat a banana most mornings – I love them, and they give me energy. But do bananas make you fat? ... and so begins the banana anxiety.

Later, quite by coincidence, I noticed this link on Twitter: 'According to a Japanese scientific research, a banana contains TNF which has anti-cancer properties. The degree of anti-cancer effect corresponds to the degree of ripeness of the fruit. In other words, the riper the banana, the better the anti-cancer quality. Eat bananas for optimum health.' Instantly I began to feel better.

The same thing happened recently with peanut butter. After I wrote my *Times* column, I received this email from a reader: 'Emma, do you like peanut butter? I challenge you to one slice, on toasted granary bread – with butter if you can manage. Eating small but tasty, nutritious snacks really helped me gain weight. Try it, and tell me it's not good?'

I thought about it. I'm always looking for good vegetarian sources of protein – and I like challenges. But peanut butter, quite apart from having the B word in it, is terribly fattening, isn't it? So I googled it: 'Peanut butter has long been shunned as high-fat and high-calorie, but it's not all bad. True, it contains 16 grams of fat per serving, but it's the heart-healthy, monounsaturated kind. Go for it.' And so I did. Crunchy peanut butter on piping hot toast.

*

Back to the supermarket queue, and my basket containing dairy, carbs, fruit and veg and no fat, and Alice's containing meat, fish and butter but no carbs. To be honest, I've sort of lost track of the rules: is it carbohydrates which make you overweight these days, raising insulin and storing glucose, or are trans-fats the demons, or is high-fibre the way to go? Do essential fats keep you slim, does protein build muscle? Is it simply the billion-dollar commercial industries peddling their theories to make us paranoid and faddy about what we eat? I'm not even talking about Atkins, Dukan or the 5:2 Diets – I'll look at these later – for now I'm interested in how we got suspicious of everyday foods like bread and milk and meat.

The first thing to say is that it's not just me and my sister: these days, food-wariness is well and truly mainstream. And the food and diet industry have jumped on this in a big way, reinforcing our uncertainties and pandering to our fears. Pret A Manger, for example, one of the UK's largest sandwich chains, sell 'No Bread Crayfish and Avocado' and a range of other bread-free lunches. They detected the carb-phobia early on, and have been doing very well out of it – I have female friends who refer to 'carb-free' days as casually as they would discuss the weather.

So are we phobic, faddy or simply ill-informed? The number of Brits currently claiming to have a food allergy or intolerance is more than one in five, with most singling out wheat as the culprit. This is an increase of 400 per cent in the past twenty years. Research conducted by Portsmouth University has shown that of all those claiming to have an allergy or intolerance, only 2 per cent actually do. In other words, millions of people have decided, or have been persuaded, that they have an allergy to certain foods. This could be a way of saying we don't like something, or it could be harmless hypochondria or fussiness. Perhaps we find it easier to mumble about a dairy-intolerance or gluten-sensitivity rather than admit 'I don't eat bread because it makes me gain weight.'

So food isn't simply a matter of fuel – it's also a personal issue. I made the choice not to eat meat or fish, fifteen years ago in Connecticut. I remember the exact moment I went vegetarian:

a barbecue beside the lake with my then boyfriend's family. His father handed me a plate of delicious food – large steak and a generous pile of chips. As I cut into the meat the blood gushed out and around the plate, soaking the chips a watery red. I decided there and then that I couldn't eat dead animals any more. But I've noticed how close this ethical vegetarianism creeps to full-on veganism, how easy it would be for my forbidden list to grow (a legacy, I'm sure, of the strict anorexic mindset). For example, I feel uneasy about eggs – they were once, almost, living chicks. If I think too long about milk from cows, hot milky liquid being pumped out of the udders, the artificial hormones required to keep the cattle producing milk, I begin to feel queasy. But I can't go there: I spent too long avoiding food groups. Plenty of vegans have healthy, balanced diets, but I know that it wouldn't be a wise choice for me.

But which of us doesn't have preferences when it to comes to food, favourite flavours or irrational phobias? These are often linked to happy associations or unpleasant experiences in the past. My best friend, for example, can't eat apples, ever since he bit into one as a child and a huge maggot crawled out. When he makes a simple sandwich, he says the tomato needs to be on top of the cheese, not underneath – apparently this affects the taste. Another friend will only eat carrots if they're sliced lengthways, rather than chopped into discs. My brother insists that M&Ms taste better in handfuls, rather than one by one. My boyfriend loves pineapple on his pizza, while I can't imagine mixing fruit with savoury – and my parents need to drink their morning tea from their special mugs or it just doesn't taste right.

My comfort food is baked beans – deeply unglamorous, I know, but I love them! Heinz claim to be the world's fourth biggest food and drink brand behind Coke, McDonald's and Nescafé so I'm clearly not the only one who likes baked beans. They're a global product like Marmite and Weetabix, one of those foods that people really love and miss when they emigrate. I just checked and discovered that they're exported to over sixty countries, including Russia and China. I've bought Heinz from dusty mini-markets in the Seychelles, on Greek islands, in gas stations in the Deep South. Magic food. As well as being a great source of vegetarian protein, they're naturally high in fibre and low in fat. I like my beans 'nude' – unadulterated – in a small can, eaten with a small silver spoon, ideally straight from the fridge. I know that many people would find cold baked beans revolting – mostly they're eaten hot, with a jacket potato, or on toast, or as part of a Full English breakfast. *Chacun à son goût.*

*

While our eating habits are deeply personal, food itself is laden with social connotations. The choices we make are quite mixed up, a combination of income, availability, preferences and personal food ideas: e.g. fresh is better than frozen; supporting local shops is a priority; large supermarkets are evil, etc. From childhood we have preferences around food and shopping, based on a range of factor such as where we grew up, our parents' income, family habits and food tastes. We differ in our feelings about 'value' brands, whether we drive to the supermarket and do one big shop a fortnight, or prefer to potter to the local shops and buy smaller amounts fresh every few days. My boyfriend relies on his Tesco online order once a week, my little sister always uses Ocado, but I quite like choosing my own fruit and veg in a real-live shop: these are just our personal choices.

When is the last time you went shopping at Lidl; when is the last time you went shopping at Waitrose? We all love a bargain – my father is quite a fan of the '4 pints of milk for £1' at Iceland

– but there is undeniably a difference in atmosphere and shopping experience. Lidl, Aldi and Iceland, for example, proclaim their cheap-deals with huge yellow stickers, whereas Waitrose and Sainsbury's opt for more discreet 'price-matching' labels. Some shoppers pursue price and convenience; others feel the moral and environmental responsibility of consumerism. A friend of mine in her sixties would never buy her fruit and veg from anywhere but the local market stalls (and yet she admits that she often finds bruised apples at the bottom of her bag).

As well as our personal quirks and habits, we're also heavily influenced by advertising and marketing, with their myriad messages about what we 'deserve'; what we're 'worth'; how the successful, happy consumer looks and eats. For large corporations, especially food producers and supermarkets, brand value is worth millions. When a brand is perceived to be tainted – recent examples include Bernard Matthews' turkey products, or Starbucks' UK tax affairs – consumers can very quickly turn against it.

As well as the basic publicity function of advertising, there's an awful lot of subliminal communication going on too. Waitrose were early adopters of artisan and provenance products: when I shop there I feel somehow more ethical. It's the same with Marks & Spencer – I know I go there for a 'treat' or for special occasions. Perhaps the higher prices make me feel less bad about abandoning the local greengrocer; perhaps it feels less like a bland supermarket.

For the big retailers, communicating a message ('Mum's gone to Iceland') or creating a sense of aspiration ('Sainsbury's: Taste the Difference') is all-important. Why else would multinational food companies spend so much on celebrities as the face of their products: from Melanie Sykes advertising Boddingtons in the 1990s, to Gary Lineker and Walkers crisps, Kerry Katona and Iceland, George Clooney and Nespresso. The marketing messages are skilful, persuasive pieces of image-crafting. Our high-street carrier bags say a lot about us.

Where we buy our food is not only based on household budgets or tastes – it can also be a lifestyle choice, as much as holidaying in Tuscany or sending your children to private school. This was highlighted recently, when a social media stunt by Waitrose went spectacularly wrong (causing general hilarity). Some PR wonk decided it would be a good idea if customers were asked to count the ways they loved the supermarket chain, completing the phrase 'I shop at Waitrose because...' and posting it on Twitter with the hashtag #WaitroseReasons.

The campaign backfired, with Waitrose finding itself repeatedly mocked as the ponce's choice. While some submitted genuine reasons, others pounced on the opportunity to mock the brand's posh image: *I shop at Waitrose because I was once in the Holloway Road branch and heard a dad say 'Put the papaya down, Orlando'*. Another tweeted: *I shop at Waitrose because I absolutely detest being surrounded by poor people*. The ridicule continued, with quips such as: *I shop at Waitrose because – don't be silly, I have servants to do that for me* and *I shop at Waitrose because darling, Harrods is just too much of a trek mid-week*.

Many tweets ridiculed the high prices at Waitrose, with one saying: *I shop at Waitrose because I think food must automatically be better if it costs three times as much*. On the *Management Today* website, Matthew Gwyther said: 'The truth of the matter is that we would all, given the money and the chance, probably shop at Waitrose. I've experienced some of the more existentially depressing moments of my life in a Tesco Express or Sainsbury's Local.' Eventually Waitrose tweeted: 'Thanks for all the genuine and funny #WaitroseReasons tweets. We always like to hear what you think and enjoyed reading most of them.'

It's hardly a PR catastrophe – I'm sure the company was delighted with the publicity generated – but it does highlight how self-aware, even self-conscious, we are as consumers. Seems I'm not the only one who feels a bit more sophisticated when my basket is filled with organic blueberries from Waitrose, rather than Basics Value bananas from Tesco.

I have female friends who now buy exclusively organic, who cook wild-farmed salmon for their toddlers, who make pesto by hand. They want their children to be healthy, and it all sounds delicious, but I think back with nostalgia to my own childhood in the 1980s. As well as home-cooked meals, we ate fish fingers and oven chips (from the freezer), or macaroni cheese, toad-in-the-hole, or bangers and mash. For afters we might have Angel Delight as a special treat, a powdered mousse pudding. Or jelly and ice cream, or just fresh fruit. We ate apples, tangerines, pears – with five children, mum was forever filling up the fruit bowl. But my parents weren't obsessive about our five-a-day. And none of my siblings or friends were unhealthy or overweight.

Mealtimes have changed out of all recognition to what the average family would have been sitting down to a hundred or even fifty years ago – and of course this isn't just about foodie fashions, fads, or social aspirations. One of the greatest determinants of what we eat has been the general affluence of the population – such as the food shortages during the two World Wars of the twentieth century – and the availability of different kinds of food. And as we travel more, an ever-wider range of European and international cuisine has found its way home with us: French, Italian and Spanish, Mexican, Thai and Vietnamese.

Despite the fact that frozen food such as vegetables often have higher levels of nutrients than fresh produce – frozen peas, for example, or berries – as they're preserved within hours of picking, many of us still disapprove of the freezer (a modern miracle). We may not like to admit it, but we do judge people on the dietary choices they make. Frozen food is a guilty secret, while fresh – ideally covered-in-earth-fresh – is king. Some people disapprove of those who feed their children 'junk food' or defrost something quick and easy; others disapprove of microwave 'ready-meals'. And as for Chinese takeaway, pizza and curries, as tasty as they are, you'd be unlikely to serve them to dinner guests.

In the last few years farmers' markets have sprung up around the country (there are more than 750 regular markets in the UK) as has the mania for buying 'local'. London's Borough Market is a hip weekend destination for aspiring, affluent foodies from miles around. Walking past the cheese stalls in Islington's Chapel Market, I'm astounded at the prices: you can buy Brie, Camembert and Stilton at half the price in Sainsbury's opposite. At my big sister's local foodie street market in Pimlico you see young children sharing gourmet chorizo rolls and handmade quiche, while their middle-class parents stock up on fresh-roasted Arabica beans, doling out twenty-pound notes at every stall. Hard not to reflect that not far away, schoolkids and adults are paying 79p for jumbo sausage rolls from Greggs the Baker.

The craze for farmers' markets comes in part from environmental concern about food miles, in part a growing desire to know where and how our food is produced. But there's no denying the class and wealth dimension to food these days; and there's more than a whiff of self-righteousness to the movement. How smug is the term 'artisan foods'? What does it even mean?

A school friend just posted this ad for her new business on Facebook: 'At the heart of *Organic* is love: love of the land, love of nature, love of the task of raising living things with respect, love of the process and the people involved in it, love of health, love of food and the flavors, smells and textures of something created with enthusiasm, care and commitment.' It sounds great – but god, so worthy.

The model-turned-farmer Liz Hurley is evangelical about her decision to eat only organic: 'I almost never eat anything from a tin or a packet... I'm passionate about home-cooked food and am convinced that eating a lot of packaged and processed food encourages weight gain. If you think about it, a homemade cake has only four ingredients: butter, eggs, sugar and flour but if you look at the ingredients list of a shop-bought cake, it can be quadruple that – and most of it stuff you don't want in your body.'

Of course we're expected to shudder at the thought of those nasty 'shop-bought' cakes. Who knows what 'stuff' it might contain – almost certainly 'stuff you don't want in your body'.

I smiled recently at this opinion piece online from *Sydney Morning Herald* writer Jacqueline Maley: 'One of the more insidious trends of the modern era... is the moral sanctity people attach to their food choices. Eating is no longer something we do for taste and energy consumption; it is a political act. The ability to select and consume biodynamic, macrobiotic, locally sourced and fully organic food is surely the greatest middle-class indulgence of our time.'

A middle-class indulgence indeed. And the foodie lifestyle is spreading. Back in 2003 the news that Liz Hurley was going into farming seemed incongruous, to say the least. What would a MAW (model-actress-whatever) know about sausage-making?

Nevertheless, she persevered, producing an organic range from her 400-acre estate in Gloucestershire, with her four Labradors, two cats, three geese, eight chickens, forty-nine cows, sixty-three sheep and eighty-two pigs. In between bringing out new bikini and beachwear lines, she gave countless interviews extolling the virtues of rural living and baking muffins on the Aga.

More recently Hurley seems to have fallen out of love with her rare-breed Gloucester Old Spot pigs, and spends a lot of time in Australia with her new man, cricketer Shane Warne.

Alex James used to be a lithe-hipped, floppy-haired sex god and bassist in the Britpop band Blur. He is now a passionate cheese-maker, food columnist for *The Sun*, and all-round gastro-snob. No longer a sex god (IMHO) he now wears tweed jackets, is married with five children, and hob-nobs with the Chipping Norton set, a group of Conservative MPs and media folk in Oxfordshire.

Gwyneth Paltrow and Sophie Dahl have also joined in, with recipe books, blogs and TV cooking programmes. Suddenly models are foodies, actresses are chefs, musicians are organic farmers. Food-as-lifestyle is well and truly here.

*

Part of the fun of getting older is nostalgia, isn't it? Remembering how much nicer, friendlier, and happier things were when you were young. We all do it – but in the case of food, I do remember things being simpler. As a teenager it was totally normal on a Saturday shopping spree with girlfriends to stop for a cheeseburger and fries. 'Fast food' didn't carry any stigma, really. I haven't been to McDonald's or Burger King since the early 1990s – and a survey of my thirty-something friends confirms the same: 'literally haven't eaten a Big Mac in decades'. These days there are clear distinctions in the convenience food market: Leon, Pret A Manger and YO! Sushi on one side, and McDonald's, Burger King and KFC on the other, and we all have our preferences. A friend of mine commented the other day that no one brings fast food into the office any more. He works in the financial sector, an all-male workplace except for two secretaries, and they all eat lunch *al desko*. 'I usually pick up a sandwich from EAT, and a smoothie, or a wrap from Starbucks with my coffee, or a salad from the juice bar downstairs.' A salad? My ultra-blokey friend? Truly this is a brave new world. Some of my colleagues bring in leftover pasta from the night before, most go to the local deli or coffee shop and buy sandwiches. But no one returns to the office with that (deliciously) smelly brown paper bag with the quarter-pounder and large fries any more.

The lunchtime options for most of us working in offices are growing all the time. Only a decade ago, if you worked in a busy town centre you might have the option of a burger chain, a supermarket, and maybe a sandwich shop or a local caff. Today, within a five-minute walk from my flat are the following: Starbucks, EAT, Pod, Leon, Pret A Manger, Caffè Nero, Abokado, itsu, You-Me-Sushi, YO! Sushi, Costa Coffee, Hummus Bros and Subway, and that's without counting the independent cafes and greasy spoons, delicatessens, corner shops and supermarkets, plus a couple of gourmet falafel vans and the uber-trendy eateries like O-Zone, Shoreditch Grind and Pizza East. OK, I'm in central London, but that's still a heck of a lot of choice. Across Britain, the average town centre now offers a wider food range than ever before, and you find wraps and smoothies available in most motorway service stations.

Food outlets and their advertisers are also clever with the lifestyle they offer us. For those of us who grew up watching American sitcoms in the 1980s and 1990s 'grabbing a coffee' is still cool. And yet there are kettles in most kitchens: we could make a cup of tea or coffee at work. I asked a friend why we waste £10 or £20 a week on Starbucks coffee – does it taste better than instant? 'For me it's part of the morning routine – I love walking into the office clutching my takeaway coffee – subliminally I'm in Manhattan, a successful young PA for a glamorous art gallery on the Upper East Side, I'm a Google entrepreneur, or Melanie Griffiths in *Working Girl*, I'm Rachel in *Friends*!' And that's so true: with their recycled cardboard cups, the satisfying paper bags with overpriced yogurt and granola for breakfast, they're cleverly selling us a more glamorous image of ourselves.

Or look at the branding of Starbucks' Refresha: a 'thirst-quenching' blend of coffee, cool lime and citrus juice. The name has been carefully chosen to convey a summery, sexy, and somehow healthy beverage. A few years ago you'd struggle to find a photograph of Britney Spears not holding her trademark iced coffee (or grande frappuccino or whatever they were calling it). We've all seen the beautiful people clutching their takeout coffee cups – it's one of those celebrity props, like an expensive handbag or a little dog.

It should be quite simple, selling sandwiches or coffee, but it's not. The big chains are hyper-aware of their own image, and careful to differentiate themselves. Pret A Manger, for example, make great play of the fact that none of their sandwiches have use-by dates; they don't need them because they're 'handmade' fresh every day. They sell only 'natural food' avoiding the 'nasties' common to their competitors, and they refer frequently to 'honest' ingredients, as if regular food preservatives were somehow criminal. EAT brands itself as The Real Food Company (as opposed to what, one wonders) and offers Miso Soup, Gourmet Wraps, Superfood Salads.

My favourite example of pretentious lifestyle food is itsu – or rather *itsu Health & Happiness!* This hip sushi chain, founded by Pret's Julian Metcalfe, recently opened a branch on the corner of my street and I'm following their progress with mirth. Each week, a new poster goes up in the window, not of their sandwiches or sushi, but black and white images of bikini-clad women laughing as they splash through the surf, or a man with a rippling six-pack catching a beach ball. This must explain why they're called itsu Health & Happiness: if you eat there, you will be young and beautiful, healthy and happy.

The menu offers *bright salads, crunchy vegetables, healthy brown rice, warming & light Asian soups, fresh sushi, skinny sandwiches, moreish mayonnaise-free sauces, rice cakes rather than cake cakes & refreshing i·tea cocktails*. The message from itsu is unequivocal: caffeine is bad, cakes are evil, sandwiches must be 'skinny' and mayo is banned! It's all about steamed fish and clean eating; even the crisps are made of air-dried seaweed.

Here's a sample of itsu's marketing (taken from their website): 'We have an absolute ban on mayonnaise. We don't sell lattes. We don't clutter our shops with cakes and cookies.' And there's more... 'We do, however, build a butterfly light kitchen in every single itsu and here we make our Eat Beautiful menu on the hour, every hour. We are utterly dedicated to butterfly light food at butterfly light prices. Big smile, small tummy... food that fills us up and makes us happy.'

Why the cutesy marketing-speak about small tummies; are we seven years old?! This is a perfect example of 'wacky-writing' popularised by Innocent Smoothies and their chummy babytalk packaging: 'We're not saying that there's anything wrong with going for a gym workout, it's just, you know, all a bit of an effort really, isn't it? If I were you, I'd just have an Innocent smoothie instead.' Pret call one of their puddings a 'Chocolate Moose'.

*

As if the food branding and advertising wasn't enough, we're also witnessing a growing television obsession with food. Some evenings we're served a wall-to-wall schedule of cookery programmes, baking competitions, inviting-guests-round-for-dinner shows, and celebrity versions of *Masterchef*. The male chefs have their macho TV shows: Jamie Oliver bashing things around the kitchen and Gordon Ramsay swearing a lot. The female foodies serve up culinary porn: Nigella Lawson in a low-cut top seductively eating spaghetti, or Sophie Dahl staring doe-eyed into the camera as she stirs a casserole. Maybe it's no wonder we're obsessed with eating, not eating, losing weight and getting fat. As well as being surrounded by food outlets when we venture outside, assailed by diet and calorie discussions with girlfriends and colleagues, we also have television and magazines shoving it down our throats. If it's bad in the UK, it's even worse in the home of obesity: the United States. On a road trip across the US last year I was amazed at the sheer quantity of food on offer: twenty or thirty different types of bread in the supermarkets, hundreds of breakfast cereals, endless diet this and low-fat that, lite and sugar-free versions. Looking at some of the morbidly obese shoppers, their trolleys stuffed with family-packs of crisps and cookies and sodas, it seemed that there was just too much choice. Lite or sugar-free this food may be, but calories are calories, and if you eat enough of it, stuffed with sweeteners, flavourings and artificial preservatives, you're going to get fat.

In the US, the traditional visit to the movies is accompanied by popcorn and hot dogs, sweets and candy, or even a full Mexican meal: nachos, tacos and melted cheese. As an American friend tells me, 'It's just what you do – buy movie tickets, visit the bathroom, choose the snacks.' (And the 2-litre bucket of soda!)

A fascinating research study in California (published in the *Journal of Personality and Social Psychology*) gave participants a randomly assigned bucket of either fresh or week-old stale popcorn and measured their consumption. They found that it didn't make any difference whether the participants were hungry or not before the film, or whether the popcorn was stale or fresh

– they still ate it. The study concluded that 'once we've formed an eating habit, we no longer care whether food tastes good'.

The multi-screen Odeon in the west London shopping centre Whiteleys offers a fine dining experience, courtesy of chef Rowley Leigh. For around £40 per head, you can enjoy a 'fillet steak hamburger royale, red mullet risotto, squid, salsify fritters and gourmet popcorn, plus lemon-grass ice cream, with waiter service and a glass of fine wine', all while watching your film. Cinema eating, like eating in front of the TV, is particularly damaging – when we don't notice what we're eating, we tend to keep going for longer. It's sort of boredom, sort of habit, this kind of screen grazing. It's not just at the cinema or in front of the TV: one can barely take a train journey without being encouraged to purchase 'hot and cold snacks and a range of beverages' from the trolley; gyms have cafes to fuel up on calories after you've exercised them off. Shopping malls have large food courts in case we get peckish between shops, airports are filled with restaurants and cafes, to fill in time before our flight.

A colleague yesterday was complaining about the prices at Heathrow's Terminal 5 champagne and oyster bar, Caviar House. My boss, a travel editor for the last twenty years, said: 'I remember when there was just one restaurant in Terminal 3.' Many new-build offices now have sparkly kitchens or on-site canteens (News International's canteen is like a gourmet restaurant) and food is rarely out of sight during the working day. Every big company I've worked for in London has Pret A Manger catering for meetings – and wherever you are in the country your informal meetings probably have some element of biscuits involved. Then there's the social element to office-food: bringing in the Marks & Spencer tubs – brownies, flapjacks, rocky road – it's just what you do, isn't it? This is a variation on bringing in a birthday cake I suppose.

In publishing, my female colleagues would regularly hold Friday 'bake-offs', bringing in lemon drizzle, carrot cake, scones which they'd made the night before. In advertising the Account Directors would bring trays of Dunkin' Donuts back from successful pitches. The women I work with now buy Reese's Pieces, cupcakes, pink Percy Pigs. If there's no cake tin on the go, one or other of the girls will have a sugar-crash and rush downstairs to Waitrose on a collective chocolate mission. The fact that they're often on tuna-only diets, or strict detox regimes, is beside the point – 'Sugar-free jelly can only get you so far,' they remind each other.

Even local boozers have become gastro-pubs, with elaborate menus replacing the traditional bag of salt and vinegar crisps. Starbucks, which used to do coffee with a few cakes on the side, now sells a wide range of sandwiches, pastries, muffins and cookies.

Another import from the US is nutritional information on food packaging. These are intended to empower us as consumers, to give us the full calorie, fat, carbohydrate and protein content of every item. While the traffic-light system of labelling (red, amber and green for unhealthy to healthy) has had some success in raising awareness, why is it that UK consumers continue to get fatter? We all know how misleading the serving sizes can be. For example I was recently sitting in the park with my friend D, and he was snacking on a bag of KP salted peanuts. According to the nutritional information, each 50 g serving contained 311 calories and 27 g of fat. But the bag was 200 g – so the entire bag contained 1,244 calories and 108 g of fat. 'Who only eats a quarter of a bag of nuts?' he reasoned.

So we have all this information alongside growing obesity levels: clearly something isn't working. We're overwhelmed with food-choice and flavour and lighter options and it's making us fat, anxious, obsessive, or all three. My colleagues can tell you the calorie content of everything: 'Banana?' one will ask – 'Large

THE MINISTRY OF FOOD

120, small, 80.' 'Pret Chocolate Moose?' '375 cals, 29 grams of fat.' Even at my very worst I never counted calories, so I find their encyclopaedic knowledge quite impressive.

*

As I'm writing about food, a tweet comes in from @quokkakat – I've never met her but she contacted me after reading *An Apple a Day*. She tweets: *Frozen yogurt shop just opened near me, reminded me of your book!* It reminds me of Salt Lake City, Utah, just over twelve months ago...

I'm a big fan of fro-yo – frozen yogurt – and I'm not the only one. It's been around in the US since the 1970s, where the market is now worth £8 billion, but in recent years the UK has also witnessed an explosion. Companies such as Pinkberry, Yuforia, For the Love of Yog, Red Mango, Lick Yogurt, Yoo Moo and Haagen-Dazs make big money out of satisfying the (predominantly female) hunger for fro-yo. The Snog bar in Covent Garden is staffed by achingly hip youngsters, with slick, flirty T-shirt slogans such as *You never forget your first snog*. Across London, South Kensington's branch of Snog is crowded with beautiful, skinny, rich teenage girls. In Kings Road it's all yummy mummies and green tea frozen yogurt.

Like bottled water and designer coffee, fro-yo thrives on its celebrity fans: Victoria Beckham, Lindsay Lohan, Paris Hilton, Nicole Kidman and the Kardashians have all been photographed with their funky tubs. And it's not just women – the actor Leonardo DiCaprio apparently installed a fro-yo machine in his office. *The Times* recently called it 'the undisputed It Food': lower in fat and calories than ice cream (due to the use of milk instead of cream), frozen yogurt seems healthy, sexy and sin-free. Of course it's not really a health food (there are many amusing blogs on this subject) but it tastes healthy and looks gorgeous: all swirled and blended, cute and colourful.

Another food-marketing success of recent years is cupcakes. Ever since Carrie Bradshaw in *Sex and the City* sat outside the Magnolia bakery with her glittery frosted mini-treat, cupcakes have been the trendiest retro nibble. Here, for example, is a tit-bit from the actress Blake Lively in the *Daily Mail*: 'To be around me, you must love food or I'm the most obnoxious person you've ever met,' she explained. 'I'm in a big cooking phase. That's all I talk about. If you went to my house and didn't know who it belonged to, you would not think it belonged to an actress. There's no memorabilia from my career, no showbizzy pictures on the wall. You would think it was the house of a cooking obsessive. I even have a special area set aside just for baking cupcakes.'

When I was a child, fairy cakes were a treat at birthday parties; now adult women are spending their weekends baking them, not for their children, but for their friends. The twenty-first century cupcake is Alice-in-Wonderland tiny and lovingly decorated with sprinkles. And with cupcake bakeries springing up all over the country they've become a lifestyle choice for grown-up-girls. Just last week a large beribboned box from the Hummingbird Bakery arrived at work. The girls squealed and fell upon the cupcakes. I don't get it.

Seems I'm not the only one: the feminist backlash against cupcakes has been swift and furious. I find the anger aroused by these pointless cute-cakes amusing. 'What frustrates me is the way cupcakes have been so completely embraced by otherwise sensible adult women,' says the food blogger Sophie Jordan. 'Glitter, heart-shaped sprinkles, pink frosting: these are the most infantilised baked goods available.' An anti-cupcakes blog rants: 'Cupcakes seem to be shorthand for some pointless version of post-feminism. Get me a real cake, like a nice bit of banana bread or a good old carrot cake. I'll leave the nausea-inducing sugar-laden sponge to the morons.'

If these bloggers find cupcakes infantilised, I wonder what they will make of 'cake pops' – the new baking craze for cakes on lollipops. Like cupcakes they're small and cute, just a bite-sized sweet treat, presumably for delicate girly appetites. Online, the US blogger Bakerella gushes: 'I'm excited to share some cute new snowman cake pops with you guys today. I made them for my friend Betty. As in Crocker. As in cra-zee!' Wince.

When it comes to male and female food, there's no doubt about the gender of cupcakes – aimed squarely at women in the same way that Yorkie bars have been aimed at men since their launch in the 1970s. Back in the 1980s toy lorries with the Yorkie bar logo were manufactured by Corgi, and television advertisements for the Yorkie bar featured manly truck drivers. In 2001, Yorkie's ad campaign caused controversy with the slogan *It's not for girls*, though they have recently rolled out a campaign that gently mocks heroic males doing tasks such as carrying in the supermarket shopping in a single trip.

And it's not only cupcakes: other sweet treats play on this irritating modern concept of 'treating oneself'. Women's magazines endlessly peddle this rubbish about 'me-time': whether it's a bubble bath and a glass of wine, or an evening out with 'the girls', or indulging yourself with a massage or a manicure. It is infantilising, I think, and unnecessary. We're grown women, running our own lives, earning our own money – we don't need silly excuses for buying or eating something pleasurable.

I remember my Liverpool Nana settling onto the couch at the end of the day in front of *Coronation Street* with her supper laid out on a tray. This would be sausages or a lamb chop with greens or potatoes, then a cream horn for pudding – and *always* a small bottle of Guinness warming by the electric fire. 'Just a little something to treat myself' she'd say, like the cat that got the cream. I loved how much pleasure it gave her. Many years on and the megabrand L'Oreal taps into this same female, slightly coy, sentiment: 'because you're worth it'. The advertising industry has long thrived on this concept of 'treating ourselves'. Even before the 1970s slogan 'naughty but nice' (coined, weirdly enough, by Salman Rushdie) they have described desserts and confectionery in terms of indulgence or sin. What used to be the sweet at the end of the meal – bread and butter pudding, say, or jam roly-poly – is now a guilty, often erotic, pleasure: remember the 'crumbliest flakiest chocolate' scene with the naked woman eating a Flake bar in the bath.

At a gastro-pub recently I was amazed at the desserts listed on the menu: vanilla bean and white chocolate panna cotta, summer berry pavlova, limoncello syllabub with crushed amaretti, chocolate truffle torte. In an English country boozer!

Aren't we all sophisticated these days? Think how rapidly the food landscape is changing – think of what you ate as a child, for your packed lunch, on family holidays, at birthday parties. These days middle-class kids are quite familiar with taramasalata, avocado or tzatziki. When I take my nieces and nephew (seven, five and two) to Starbucks they're catered for with babyccinos, where the barista froths up some milk in an espresso-sized cup. They may be young but they have opinions on different types of pasta – conchiglie versus penne – and they confidently eat food which I'm sure my siblings and I would have prodded suspiciously as children (e.g. risotto, granola, polenta). I still surprise myself with my new love of couscous – as a child I'd never even heard of it.

A friend in her fifties had me in stitches recently reminiscing about the first appearance of quiche – they pronounced it 'kwich' – in her East Midlands family home. 'It was a pie made of egg.

With bits of bacon in it.' Pizza was also foreign, and rather glamorous. Slightly older, my godmother Rita remembers the austerity and rationing of the post-War years. It was wholesome, filling food – what we would call classic British cuisine these days – roasts, steak and kidney pie, spotted dick, bread and butter pudding. Food designed to fill you up. Certainly no low-carbing.

It's hard to appreciate how scarce food really was. Rita tells me about visiting the British Restaurants with her mother – 'a sort of genteel soup kitchen for those who were really hard up.' She showed me the rationing books which her mother left when she died: it was quite a wake-up call for those of us born into post-War plenty. Here, from the Home Sweet Home Front website, is an example of an adult's typical week's ration in 1943, halfway through the Second World War:

3 pints of milk
¾ lb – 1 lb meat
1 egg (or 1 packet of dried eggs every 2 months)
3–4 oz cheese
4 oz bacon and ham
2 oz tea
8 oz sugar
2 oz butter
2 oz cooking fat
+ 16 points a month for other rationed foods (usually enough points to buy one can of tinned meat or fish) subject to availability.

These weekly rations were stretched with the help of un-rationed extras like bread (not rationed until after the war), cereal, potatoes, offal, fruit and vegetables.

I try to compare this to me and my sisters and girlfriends with our elaborate food intolerances, carb-avoidance and gluten-free wheat-free-fussiness. As someone who spent years not allowing myself to eat, I feel sort of ashamed. I remember what Rita said; 'There wasn't any choice – you'd be grateful for potatoes, a bit of meat, some fat, whatever they had.'

Perhaps if we had to spend our time simply finding enough food to get by, there would be no time for obesity. Or slimming, for that matter. I freely admit that anorexia is a disease associated with affluence, and research backs this up: in developing countries where food is scarce, anorexia is almost unheard of. (It does exist in these countries but is often linked to impulses of religious purity and self-denial rather than concerns around body shape or weight.) And what about bulimia? The concept of literally flushing vast amounts of food down the lavatory would have seemed terribly wasteful during those years of war and rationing.

*

For any of us born in the late twentieth century it's hard to get our heads around genuine food scarcity. It's even hard to imagine a world where bananas and pineapples were a rarity. Right now, with a single click at Tesco online I can order lychees, Asian pears or physalis berries, or any number of unusual products that I can hardly identify. I could nip to the corner shop and spend £5 on a carton of Vita Coco, 'an all-natural, super-hydrating, fat-free, cholesterol-free, nutrient-packed, potassium-stacked, mega-electrolyte coconut water'.

In the summer of 2012 the *Evening Standard* declared 'the capital has gone crazy for coconuts'. A company called Coco Face began importing fresh Thai coconuts for hip young Londoners at pop-up street markets and food festivals. They served them with a straw inside to suck up the juice, or split open to eat the flesh, or as cocktails with white rum and a twist of lime. Other entrepreneurs exploited the tropical fruit for coconut and cinnamon popcorn, and toasted coconut ice cream. Selfridges saw a 100 per cent increase in sales of a new coconut milk yogurt called Coyo. Converts raved about the antiviral, antibacterial, anti-inflammatory and anti-oxidant properties of coconut water.

So we have easy access to exotic cuisine from every corner of the globe; we're overwhelmed by nutritional advice and information; spoilt for choice. Why should this affluence cause us to over-eat or under-eat? Why should it make us so dissatisfied with our own bodies, and create an obsession with thin? It has, I think, caused a crisis of confidence. When everything is available, nothing is ever enough.

We've all stood in front of rows of dresses in a shop, unable to find the right one for a party or wedding. We all recognise that jaded feeling on Boxing Day, when you look around at the Christmas presents, clothes, and discarded wrapping paper and realise you don't need any of it. We've all logged off the Internet feeling burned out from hours spent browsing, dazed by all the products and opinions out there – and it's increasingly hard ever to go offline. We can access TV and radio programmes anytime, anywhere, on our iPhones, iPads, tablets, and countless other 'smart' devices. Google are talking confidently about implanting computer chips in our brains soon enough. When you consider the near-infinite range of lifestyle, entertainment and cosmetic options available, it's no wonder we don't know what we really want.

This limitless choice, particularly in nutritional terms, seems to have left us less satisfied, not more. We throw away more rotten produce year on year: stuff we buy and can't be bothered to use, or didn't want in the first place.

We are growing obese while barely stopping to taste the food. Just as tourists view the wonders of the world from behind their camera-phones instead of their own eyes, we're just going through the motions, always missing the real experience. It's a Western luxury of course, all this abundance, and it leaves us unsatisfied. Like children with too many toys and not enough boundaries, we keep demanding and consuming more, more, more.

And the brave new world, highly visual and hyper-connected, only makes matter worse. We're bombarded with digital images from morning till night, many of us literally unable to turn off our smart phones until after we turn out the lights. Constant comparison with others (more attractive or successful) leads to personal dissatisfaction, and a profound sense of insecurity. If you don't already feel fat and ugly today, just flick through the celebrity magazines for a quick fix.

And if you're still fat or ugly or old – why aren't you fixing it? When you consider the so-called miracle diets, cosmetic and nutritional quick-fixes on offer, it's no wonder so many of us are confused about what to eat, what to weigh, and how to look. After all, if some women are impossibly slim and beautiful, shouldn't you be too?

Chapter 2

THE MINISTRY OF FAT

Let me tell you about my phobia of fat.

In the worst days of anorexia, I would rather have slammed my hand in a door than spread butter on a slice of toast. I would have chosen to jump off a ten-foot diving board rather than add whipped cream to my black coffee. I would have preferred to eat an insect than drink a full-fat milkshake. My attitude is a lot more chilled out nowadays, but I remember this intense fear of fat all too well.

A few years ago during my weight-gain process, my boyfriend bought me a large chunk of Cheddar cheese and begged me to try it. It took several weeks of dodging it every time I opened the fridge before I made myself lay a thin slice of cheese onto plain brown bread. And eat it.

Recently in the supermarket, I saw a woman putting a couple of square blocks of 'lard' in her shopping basket and I was appalled. I don't know what the lard was for – baking a cake? Cooking a chicken? The threat of fat is everywhere, I thought, why would she consciously seek it out? Had she never heard the word 'lardy'?

I remember as a child, mum would tell us about her childhood meals – one of them was a Liverpool speciality, or perhaps a Northern speciality, called 'bread and dripping'. It's a sort of butty – goose fat spread thickly on bread – and I used to think it sounded quite tasty. I can't imagine eating it now.

Recently my Irish friend J called me while she was halfway through cooking an anniversary meal for her husband. I asked what she was making, and she mentioned the starter was a shellfish bisque. She said, 'and then I add cream to the soup...' I didn't understand this, and questioned her more closely: 'Why the cream?' 'It thickens it up something gorgeous. And of course it tastes so good,' she replied. The idea that you would add cream to soup – or butter to bread – or mayonnaise to a salad sandwich – is where I get stuck. Of course it improves the taste – I love the taste of cream, butter or cheese as much as the next person, although I can barely remember it – but that you would *willingly* add fat to food – seems insane.

The concept of flavour is not wasted on me: I know that regular hummus tastes better, and is probably healthier, than low-fat versions; I understand that fat-free yogurt is full of sugar and other flavourings to compensate for the lack of fat. I agree with my sister when she says that skimmed milk 'tastes like grey water' (and I keep promising myself I will switch to semi-skimmed). I remember happy days in France, tearing open a warm baguette and spreading it with butter, freshly churned from the cows in the field, or a slice of melting Brie or Camembert: there is nothing unhealthy about that. I remember Sunday afternoons with my sisters and brothers, all piled into the playroom, listening to the Pop Chart Top 40 countdown, sharing Maltesers or Curly-Wurlies or Toblerone.

Rationally, I know that fat is an important part of a balanced diet. We need fat as we need protein and carbohydrates. I understand that fats are essential for healthy hair, for glowing skin – I have experienced the effects of malnourishment and fat deficiency. I found out the hard way that when your body has zero fat, your reproductive system shuts down, your breasts and hips and curves disappear, your libido hits the floor.

I accept the need to consume some healthy fats – those found in nuts, olive oil and avocados, for example. But much as I enjoy these foods, and know they're doing me good, I still have to fight a constant battle with myself not to avoid them. Because fat is the thing I fear above all else.

*

This is the way I feel about fat in food. However, fat as body-shape seems quite different. It interests me: I wonder what it would be like to become very large.

Of course 'fat' is a very loaded word. I try to use it literally, to describe the deposits of fatty layers under the skin and around organs – but look, already that word 'fatty' sounds judgemental. The facts are simple: our bodies are made up of lean tissue and adipose or fat tissue. Lean tissue is composed of muscle, bone and organs. Fat tissue is composed of three different categories: essential fat, storage fat and non-essential fat. A 'fat' person simply has a large amount of excess flesh, but they carry so much more than that. As a society we're ashamed of being fat, afraid of getting fat – and horrified at some of the immense fatness we see around us today.

We're in a bit of a mess when it comes to fat, I think. We know there is a problem, but we don't know how to approach it or what to do about it. Recent proposals to outlaw the use of the term 'fat' in a medical context don't offer a solution either, igniting accusations of political correctness gone mad etc. But are the words 'stout' or 'corpulent' or 'obese' any better?

From the other end of the spectrum I'm aware that whatever I write will be wrong. I'm skating on thin ice: what could be more irritating than a thin person calling another person fat? And yet – for a moment – think about how we describe thinness: skinny, scrawny, angular, stick-insect, emaciated, bony, skeletal, lollipop-head, underfed, anorexic. Such terms are batted about in the media quite casually, without the caution we must now use in our references to fat. A recent headline in the Saturday *Times* magazine proclaimed: 'Curvy is the New Skinny'. Note the tactful use of 'curvy' and the tactless use of 'skinny'. I happen to find the term 'skinny' offensive, but of course that's foolish. *You're lucky to be thin*, people think, rolling their eyes.

But I'll try to explain how it feels. Five years ago, when I worked in publishing, we had our weekly commissioning meetings every Wednesday morning. Around twenty of us would gather in the boardroom, from commissioning editor up to director level, to present new titles and discuss whether they should be signed up. There would be tea, coffee and several platters of pastries along the boardroom table. A senior colleague – a lovely women in her fifties – would always urge me to have a croissant, loudly and publicly. She would prod me in the side, in a friendly manner, while commenting: 'Look, she's nothing but skin and bone!' or 'We need to feed you up!'

The fact that I was deeply anorexic at the time is irrelevant. She was drawing attention to my size in a way that would have been unacceptable – unthinkable – for me to do about a larger person. I felt undermined in front of my colleagues, I felt deeply humiliated. I never minded presenting in those meetings, but I dreaded the awkwardness over the pastries. Imagine, for a moment, if I had done the same to her, or any of the other plus-sized women in the room. Imagine if I'd pulled her croissant away and said 'Ooh you're looking a bit obese, don't think you really need to eat that do you!'

There are a million reasons why it was OK for her to act that way, and not OK for me – that she cared about me and wanted to mother me, she was trying to tempt or encourage me, that she didn't realise I had a serious eating disorder, that she was worried about me, or simply that she hadn't thought about it – I understand all that. But it comes down to the same thing: being thin is desirable, whereas being fat is not.

And there are plenty of excuses made for being overweight, ranging from glands to genes to heavy bones. Here is the journalist Lydia Slater, writing in the *Daily Mail*, attributing her size to the influence of the people close to her: '... given I normally eat dinner with a BBQ-mad husband and a chocoholic teenage boy, it's no surprise that I pile on the pounds and have to work out daily to fit into my dresses... According to researchers at the University of Birmingham, we are subconsciously influenced by the eating habits of those around us.'

So we blame our size on anything but our own behaviour. We tiptoe around fatness, calling it curvy or ample or hourglass-shaped. Women's magazines play a devious game of peddling thinness at all costs, while simultaneously preaching self-acceptance. Even as they're advising us how to lose weight, cut calories and burn fat, they're reminding us to love the shape we're in. They worship the slender, and pretend to glorify the fuller-figure, holding up the singer Adele as a role model for 'real' women (when she's just a great singer).

No wonder we get so tied up in knots about size. But what is it, really, which makes fat such a taboo? My friend R, who's a normal size 12–14, was candid when I quizzed her on this: 'Skinny-minnies make you feel envious, even sort of suspicious; fat friends are good, you can be comfortable around them. And you can eat with them.'

*

It's difficult to discuss fat neutrally when there is so much fear and misinformation around. The warnings are well-rehearsed: that obesity is a ticking time-bomb; that children are facing a future of chronic weight-related illness. And yet we've never been more obsessed with joining gyms and going on diets and buying healthy foods. It's hard to work out what to believe. Some days one sees a lot of overweight people, other days the warnings of an obesity epidemic seem completely groundless. Right now, for example, in a cafe in Islington, North London: there are three businessmen sitting near me, all slim; two women, one quite overweight, one slender.

But that's an entirely unscientific survey. If I was sitting in a cafe in Nottingham the story might be very different: the East Midlands has the highest average BMI at 28.9, followed by Scotland with an average BMI of 28.4. (BMI is calculated by dividing weight in kilograms (kg) by height in metres squared – a BMI above 25 is defined as overweight and above 30 is defined as obese.) Seven out of ten people in cities like Leicester, Derby and Nottingham are on the borderline between overweight and obesity. London has the lowest body mass in the UK, although the average BMI of 26.1 is still classed as overweight.

In recent years, the standard Body Mass Index measurement has been discredited as a blunt instrument, because it takes no account of the fact that abdominal fat, the so-called 'apple-shape', tends to be more dangerous than fat around the bottom and thighs, the 'pear-shape'. Nor does BMI take into account the fact that healthy muscle weighs more than unhealthy fat. For example, even though many body builders have only 10 per cent body-fat, a BMI calculator would give them an 'overweight' result. A BSI (Body Shape Index) which combines BMI and waist circumference, has been introduced as a possible alternative to BMI.

Individual health is clearly influenced by a range of socioeconomic and geographical factors within the UK, and also globally. Compared to the rest of Europe, in the UK we have higher than average obesity rates: 22 per cent, compared to an average obesity rate in the European Union of 15.5 per cent. Globally, America has traditionally been the nation of the overweight, and some of the scariest statistics come from there:

- Over 58 million Americans are overweight
- Over 40 million Americans are obese
- Over 3 million Americans are morbidly obese
- More than 80 per cent of Americans do not engage in adequate physical activity
- More than one quarter of all Americans are considered to be 'completely sedentary'

Where America goes the rest of the world follows, so we cannot ignore these statistics. Empirically we know there are more fat people around than ten or twenty years ago. I was surprised, on a recent trip to Cape Town, at how many South Africans were extremely overweight. Nowhere else in Africa have I seen this: proof, of course, that obesity is a disease of affluence. As well as being a sign of affluence, paradoxically, it's also a sign of social deprivation. This is important to remember: for all our talk of food and lifestyle 'choices', for many it may not be a choice at all. Groups from economically disadvantaged backgrounds tend to have less access to fresh food, and less knowledge and time to prepare healthy meals from scratch. They may rely on cheaper convenience food, or simply not have the education or resources to make nutrition a priority. Evansville, Indiana, was crowned in 2011 as 'America's fattest town'. The undertakers now stock super-coffins designed to hold corpses weighing up to 50 stone – and the average age of these corpses is getting younger. In the UK too, the National Health Service has been forced to increase the size of operating tables, wheelchairs, beds and hoists, to cope with wider, heavier patients. Clearly we are getting fatter, but how bad is it; can these statistics, collated on the BBC website, really be true?:

- 70 per cent of men and 63 per cent of women in the UK are overweight or obese. *(Source: Royal College of Physicians/ Faculty of Public Health)*
- 60 per cent of men, 50 per cent of women and 25 per cent of children will be obese by 2050 if no action is taken. *(Source: Royal College of Physicians/Department of Health)*
- Obesity reduces life expectancy on average by nine years. Obesity accounts for 30,000 deaths a year in the UK. *(Source: UK National Audit Office)*
- For each additional can of fizzy (sugar-sweetened) drink that a child consumes every day their risk of obesity increases by 60 per cent. *(Source: The Lancet)*
- One in five children in Britain eat no fruit at all. *(Source: National Diet and Nutrition Survey)*
- The prevalence of obesity in England has more than tripled in the last twenty-five years. *(Source: National Obesity Observatory)*

Are these reputable journals, scientists and health experts just trying to scare us? And if so, why? We've been hearing these dire warnings for years now and they aren't helping. Back in 2007, the Health Secretary Alan Johnson said that the obesity epidemic was a crisis on a scale with climate change. Dr Colin Waine, chair of the National Obesity Forum, said 'Children are likely to die before their parents.' Such statements make great headlines but are not conducive to rational debate.

On the other side, the arguments are equally problematic: claims that there is nothing wrong with being fat, that the overweight live longer than the underweight, even claims that the health warnings about obesity are simple fattism.

The truth seems to lie somewhere in the middle. Being slightly overweight, like being slightly underweight, is unlikely to cause significant health problems. While the overall weight of the population *is* increasing, with men weighing around half a stone more than they did in 1993, there is no concrete evidence that we're facing an inexorable rise in obesity. Nothing is inexorable, certainly not getting fat – we can be more active and eat less junk food. Just as women used to smoke and drink alcohol throughout pregnancy, not realising the harm it was causing to their babies, and now routinely give up both cigarettes and booze, so we have the choice about continuing to gain weight as a population.

And surely that's the point. Among all the frightening statistics, the social stigma of being fat, we sometimes forget that it carries major health risks. The overweight and obese are at an increased risk for many diseases and conditions including:

- High blood pressure/hypertension
- High cholesterol
- Type 2 diabetes
- Coronary heart disease
- Stroke
- Gall-bladder disease
- Osteoarthritis
- Sleep apnoea and respiratory problems
- Some cancers (endometrial, breast, and colon)

There are serious consequences to excessive consumption. And yet we still can't have a rational debate about the health implications, because obesity is an issue fraught with fear and shame. We don't dare to talk about the simple mobility issues: how does it feel to be too fat to run for a train; what's it like in hot weather, when your thighs are chafing together; is it really tiring to carry excess weight around on your body every day? Some brave bloggers and writers have tackled this subject, but it remains taboo for most of us. As Jess, a blogger from Canada, puts it: 'If you ever mention needing to lose weight, or having to shop in the plus-size department, people look awkward and look away. It becomes your job not to make people uncomfortable, not to talk about it, not to push it.'

In my writing about anorexia I described the physical experience, because I believe people need to know. It's important to understand extreme emaciation – how your tailbone sticks out so you can barely sit on a wooden chair, how your limbs ache from lying in bed with no cushioning, how you bruise easily, and feel cold pretty much constantly. How your ribs and your hips and your shoulder-blades become this weird, coat-hanger arrangement of clashing bones. Having been angular, hard-bodied and sharp for so long, I sometimes wonder what it's like to be pillowy-soft and fleshy.

The health risks of being fat are increasingly eclipsed by the cosmetic issues. Shocking images and 'weight-loss battles' are sensationalised by the media, and there is so much nonsense around miracle diets and cosmetic surgery that we don't stop to question if or why fat is undesirable. From what we read and watch, it is easy to assume that fat is inherently ugly, and therefore bad; thin is inherently beautiful, and therefore good.

*

A few weeks ago I was discussing the taboo of fat over a coffee with the author and nutritionist Ian Marber. Later he emailed me this thought experiment from his book, *How Not to Get Fat*:

Imagine that it's a warm sunny day and you are sitting in the garden of country pub, next to the river. It's a Sunday, and you and your boyfriend/girlfriend/husband/wife/partner are with a few close friends having just had lunch and a couple of glasses of wine and are enjoying the last of it sitting in the shade.

In the near distance is the car park, and you happen to glance over towards it as a sleek car drives up. You recognise it to be one of your favourites, something you have promised yourself that one day you will own. The roof is down and the bodywork is gleaming in the sunshine; you can hear sophisticated jazz music emanating from the car as glides crisply into a parking space, the engine is switched off and the door opens and...

Now stop.

Take a few seconds and picture the type of person who you can see getting out of the car. Think about how old they might be, what they might be wearing...

Back to the gleaming car... and out steps the driver, well dressed, glossy... and fat. Not 'can't leave the house fat' but undoubtedly big, 'Florida theme park' large.

Did you imagine that? Bet you didn't.

You see, the car is cool. Being fat isn't. The two don't go together. In fact, most things that are cool don't look right when worn, carried or even driven by a fat person.

Marber himself has no personal antipathy to fat, nor does he judge people on their size; he is making a wider social point. His simple thought exercise reminds us how thin is linked with beauty, desirability, riches and success. The lean, athletic young business person getting out of the sports car, the goddess laughing in the sunshine with her perfect husband and baby, the gorgeous woman gliding into the wine bar, all tanned limbs, glowing skin and glossy hair – they're always slim aren't they;

effortlessly, naturally slim. (Can there be two more unjust words than 'naturally' and 'slim'!)

It is hard, when faced with these types, not to feel inadequate: short and stumpy and stout. I think, as a society, we're fascinated with physical perfection: it's rare and absolutely breathtaking. Even though most of us will never look anything like this – losing weight won't transform you into an Amazonian stunner, after all – we sense that fat is part of the problem. We generate so much misery and self-hatred by telling ourselves that our bodies don't look right, blaming everything on the unwanted five or ten or twenty pounds of body-fat. Because even though being fat increases the risk of all the diseases I've just listed, that's not why we diet. We diet because being fat is wrong and socially incorrect and lumpen. It's not cool.

I don't have the answers but I do know this: trying to get thin and failing is a colossal waste of time and effort and money. The pointless diets, the unvisited gym, the daily acts of self-sabotage... You know the thought process – 'I'm alone and unattractive so what's the point in going to that Spinning class'; 'I've wrecked my diet already so I might as well finish off the packet of chocolate Hob-Nobs'. You hate yourself physically, so you hate yourself mentally: failing becomes a self-fulfilling prophecy. But the health consequences of extreme fatness are real.

From my point of view, facing up to the health consequences really helped. I wasted more than a decade struggling with the mental twists and turns of anorexia. I was utterly trapped in a labyrinth of fear and control and starvation... it was only in the last few years, when I found a *health* reason to recover – my fertility – that I began to make progress. In therapy I talked endlessly and earnestly about gaining weight (as fat people talk about losing weight and the diet they're starting tomorrow) but the fact was, I still wasn't eating. While I was underweight my periods would not come back. It was only when I turned thirty and was faced with the reality of lifelong infertility that I realised something had to change. No, *I* had to change. I had to stop talking and start eating.

Perhaps, if we reframe the whole debate around fat, if we devote the same amount of time we put into detesting our appearance into worrying about our physical health, we might start to get somewhere.

I know it's easier than it sounds. I know that, despite having come close to death, I would still choose battling anorexia over battling obesity. No one wants to be fat. Everyone wants to be thinner.

*

Lots of people nowadays are too greedy. People think 'I must have a cupcake.' What do you mean you must? You'll get fat, you fool. People are too fat because they eat all the stuff in front of them. They think, 'I want a bit of choccie', and you think, 'No, don't have it you fool.'

In November 2012, the actress Joanna Lumley expressed outspoken views on why people get fat. A former model herself, and much admired for her beauty, she said that 'lettuce' was the secret to keeping her slim figure, even in her sixties. She also said that counting calories and going on diets was pointless. 'People don't need dieting books. They should just stop eating so much. There is nothing else to be said.'

Fortunately, most of us aren't as blunt as Joanna Lumley on the question of fat – but her comments are interesting. Is it as simple as she makes out: that overweight people simply 'eat all the stuff in front of them'? Is there really 'nothing else to be said'?

I want to understand why we feel the way we do about thin and fat. Clearly the connotations are very different – think about a thin person eating and a fat person eating. If we can be honest, and abandon political correctness for a moment, most of us naturally make assumptions about people based on their size. We assume that thin people must be more: controlled; abstemious; active; discerning; detached; restrained. These are mostly admirable qualities. And that fat people must be more: greedy; slothful; gluttonous; selfish; lazy. These are mostly negative qualities.

I should make it clear, I don't think of fat people in these terms, but as a society, we undeniably associate fat with greed. Being overweight is a highly visual condition. Other factors can affect body weight, such as metabolism and genetics, but on the whole, fat people eat more and move less than thin people. With the rare exception, the 'large boned' argument is specious (you don't see overweight people in famines). But the reasons for, and the experience of, being fat are far more complex than simply: 'I must have a cupcake'. Fat doesn't just attract social disapproval – it is even portrayed as sinful. There are unfortunate parallels between obesity and the seven deadly sins: wrath, greed, sloth, pride, lust, envy, and gluttony. I was fascinated by a sermon I found online, delivered by an American pastor (who is himself obese). Having discussed the other sins, he comes to the sin of gluttony.

...Well, if you or I have problems with the other six sins in this series, if we have problems with pride, anger, envy, greed, sloth or lust then other people might not know about our problem.

But those of us who are overweight are immediately and conspicuously visible. We have no place to hide.

What is gluttony? It is an excessive, insatiable desire for food that disrupts our relationship with ourselves, with others and with God. Like the other deadly sins, gluttony is a distortion of a good gift of God. Eating is one of God's good gifts. But gluttony distorts this pleasure and turns it into a compulsion. Gluttony is something that controls us. We don't control it.

... Eating, in and of itself is a good thing. What is more enjoyable than a big Sunday dinner or a church potluck, where there is far more than anyone could possibly eat? Why then would the early church fathers put gluttony on the list of the Seven Deadly Sins? Gluttony is something we joke about...

All the overweight people I know already despise their fatness and suffer terribly because of their lifestyle of overeating. I'd like to think that gluttony is the least serious of the Seven Deadly Sins. Gluttony is simply another addiction. That's all. It's an addiction to food...

(Pastor Glenn Woodson, Holbrook United Methodist Church,
Livingston, Montana)

I identify with what this pastor says about having 'no place to hide'. I can't understand how he feels when he eats and keeps on eating, long after he is actually hungry, way beyond the point of satiety. But I know the experience of feeling that one's private pain is on display on one's own body, of being looked at, of feeling horribly conspicuous. His sermon is self-aware; he admits his own gluttony and doesn't make excuses for his weight. It made me think about myself, and whether the person I am has made me thin, or whether being thin made me into the person I am: reserved, intensely private, wary. And I wonder for the first time, painfully, whether anorexia made my personality shrink too. This is paradoxical, but I don't think that external body-size correlates with what's going on inside. Because I'm thin and I've always felt greedy.

*

Gluttony or not, being overweight isn't really a deadly sin. Nevertheless, weight is a difficult issue to confront, and we're a long way from an open discussion of fat. The more widespread the obesity problem, it seems, the more we tiptoe around it. In May 2012 a parliamentary report on body image advocated the use of 'weight-neutral language'. This is part of a growing movement to get doctors and other health professionals to stop using words such as 'overweight' and 'obese'. The MPs concluded that the terms have a negative impact on body image and self-esteem, and called for doctors to 'promote broader health and lifestyle messages' instead.

Draft guidance issued by the National Institute for Health and Clinical Excellence said those who were obese should merely be encouraged to get down to a 'healthier weight'. Not everyone in the Health Service agrees – many doctors have called it political correctness gone mad. In 2010 the Public Health Minister for England, Anne Milton, argued that GPs should continue to use the word 'fat' with their patients as it was more likely to motivate them to lose weight.

I'd say there's nothing wrong with politeness: there seems little justification for calling someone 'fat' to their face, especially not in a medical setting. But being overly sensitive in the use of terminology carries its own dangers. If we avoid confronting the obesity problem, if doctors don't feel able to advise patients to lose weight, we may end up masking what is a real health crisis. Not calling fat 'fat' may even encourage a worrying trend for fat denial. It's well-known that very thin people with eating disorders tend to over-estimate their own weight and shape. Now we're starting to see that many fat people misjudge their bodies too.

In April 2012 I read an interesting *New York Times* blog by the journalist Tara Parker-Pope. She began with her own experience: 'As I was walking through the gym the other day, I caught a glimpse of an overweight woman across the room. But then I did a double take, and then another. The woman was me – I had seen my own reflection in a distant mirror and, for a split second, hadn't recognized myself.'

Parker-Pope then reports on a study from the University of Illinois, in which nearly 4,000 young men and women in Mexico were asked to estimate their body size, in categories ranging from underweight to obese. People in the normal weight range selected the correct category about 80 per cent of the time, but 58 per cent of overweight people incorrectly described themselves as normal weight. Among the obese, 75 per cent placed themselves in the overweight category, and only 10 per cent accurately described their body size.

So rather than getting worried about fatness, we may be entering what the journalist calls a 'collective state of denial' about how fat we really are. It's a delicate issue. Personally I don't have the balls to ask any fat friends the questions I could easily ask of thin friends: How do you feel about your body? What do you see when you look in the mirror? What does it feel like to be fat? (Could *you* ask a fat acquaintance those questions?)

I contacted a woman called Sindy through a Fat Acceptance website in the US. She is 5 foot 10 inches and weighs 35 stone 10 lb (around 500 lb). She was friendly and open, and very happy to discuss her size with me. She emailed: 'I've been heavy all of my life. I've come to love the way I look. I'm part of the Fat Acceptance community, which encourages women to accept their bodies whatever their weight, and not to buy into the culture of diet and shame.'

Her positivity is refreshing, but we can't ignore the serious health risks. The Fat Acceptance movement is highly controversial, and by any measure, 35 stone is a dangerous weight to subject the human body to. While I admire the ability of a woman who is able to withstand such intense societal pressures to look a certain way,

I also believe that there is a level of self-deception here too. I don't think she's disgusting or greedy, but I do think she's probably in some sort of turmoil. Extremes of any sort, from very underweight to very overweight, are physically stressful for the body. And they usually mask quite a lot of inner distress as well.

*

Why do people get fat? It's clear that over-eating is not as simple as just needing more calories than other people, the way an athlete or a mountaineer will require more fuel. Over-eating, just like under-eating, is more likely to be an avoidance or replacement activity, a way of burying pain or anxiety, to avoid facing up to the real problems in our lives. In that sense, there *are* emotional or psychological drivers for needing or wanting more food. It may become a substitute for something else which is missing: respect, fulfilment, happiness. Food is there when nothing else is, it's a reassurance, a crutch, and bingeing numbs you, just like starving. For me, not eating was a way of exerting control when everything seemed to be out of control. Things go wrong, love fails, jobs drive you crazy, people die, what can you rely on? Losing weight was at times the only certainty.

I know that getting very thin was, for me, a way of disappearing. Does getting fat work in the same way, I wonder?

Magazine and newspapers have a permanent obsession with the changing body shape of female celebrities. Any woman who loses or gains weight in the public eye is considered fair game. So when a famously fat woman loses a large amount of weight – or even a curvy woman loses a moderate amount of weight – there is the sense that they're somehow letting the side down. This has happened with Dawn French, with Sophie Dahl, and the TV chef Nigella Lawson. Whether they like it or not, these curvier women are elected as successful role models by the media; when they lose weight, they're decried as hypocrites. This does not happen with men. During 2012 the actor and comedian James Corden lost five stone. The media coverage concentrated on Corden's vitality, how trim and healthy he was looking. Charles Saatchi, Nigel Lawson and Stephen Fry have also lost large amounts of weight in the public eye, without the value judgements. Simply put, journalists find it easier to separate a man's weight from his intelligence, his abilities, his intrinsic worth as a person. They don't blame their weight loss on a 'tragic break-up' or pry into their private lives; they don't demand their 'diet secrets' or pursue them round the local park with cameras.

The scrutiny on women in the public eye is intense, and it's not just models or athletes. Even those whose physical appearance is irrelevant are judged – look at female comedians for example. Perhaps we expect funny women to be fat, or fat women to be funny: think Hattie Jacques, Roseanne Barr, Jo Brand.

Dawn French is a cautionary tale. Interrogated about her body in a 2009 interview she said: 'I can honestly say that [being overweight] doesn't bother me, though I do worry that I'll get so comfortably fat that I won't be able to walk any more. Sometimes I'll get out of bed and think, "Oooh, I need to do some exercise" – but that's probably about once a year, if that. I think the medical term for my condition is "body blindness". I may ultimately regret not looking after myself more, and plenty of people would line up to tell me that, but it doesn't concern me.'

Then in 2012 she went on a radical diet, cutting out potatoes, pasta, bread and chocolate. Even after losing what she calls her 'lovely blubber', going from 19 stone to less than 12 stone, she refused to concede that thinner is better. 'I've never disliked myself, and my weight has had nothing to do with my self-esteem. I still refuse to dislike my old body.' It's difficult to know how to interpret her words and actions – and frankly it's none of our business. But there is something at the heart of all this: do larger role models have the right to lose weight, or are they selling out? Do we feel betrayed?

Just a few months after Dawn French lost all that weight, more stories appeared ('Curse of the Yo-yo Diet?') reporting that she had regained the weight. Of course the diet-police gleefully analysed their unflattering paparazzi shots, concluding that she was losing the 'battle of the bulge'. A reminder that when it comes to the media, you can't win: if you sell your diet success to them (or even if you don't) they own you.

Wherever Dawn French settles, she very much fits the stereotype of the female comedian. Where thin women are often characterised as seductive, humourless, miserable (think Posh Spice), fat women are characterised as jolly beer-drinkers, a laugh to be around, one of the lads.

So is there a link between fat and comedy? In 2012 the comedian Miranda Hart spoke about her efforts to slim down: 'The reason I'm set on losing weight is that I'm not naturally this big, I'm naturally lean. When I put on weight, I feel like this isn't me, this isn't right. I feel like I'm wearing a fat suit.' She admits that her main downfall is her love of food: 'I've just got such a big appetite' – and satirises her own greediness to wonderfully comic effect. In her 2012 autobiography *Is It Just Me?* she draws up a Beauty Manifesto, in which she explains her hatred of the spa, hairdressers and all things grooming-related. I found myself laughing out loud as she talked about the typical spa experience: 'A trim woman in a uniform will lead you into a little interrogation suite, where she'll quiz you on your diet, exercise and skincare habits. You'll lie through your teeth and claim that you jog five times a week, enjoy yoga, avoid sugar... the trim woman will look at you sceptically as you stand and your Emergency Maltesers fall out of your pocket onto the floor.'

Nevertheless Hart finds comments about her weight and appearance hard to deal with: 'As a woman, it seems you can't just be a comedian, you're always classed as something else too, whether that's "beautiful", "pint-sized", "larger-than-life" or in my case "the giraffe"...'

Fat and thin have more in common than we think, but neither state is funny. Whether it's physical, a layer of 'lovely blubber' to hide behind, or psychological, shutting out the world and keeping sexual interest at bay, fat can be a defence mechanism. It may be that comedy is a way of pre-empting the ridicule: I'll make jokes about my weight so that you don't.

Hart's comments about being called 'the giraffe' are interesting – at 6 foot 1, she is much taller than the average woman. It is often this experience of feeling like an outsider which drives and inspires comedians: looking unusual, or being very tall or small, or being somehow different: think of the eccentric Ken Dodd, or tiny Ronnie Corbett or cross-dressing Dame Edna Everage. The Iranian-born British comedian Shappi Khorsandi frequently satirises her experiences as an ethnic minority. (She also refers to being the fat kid at school.) My friend P does stand-up comedy on the amateur circuit and always opens with a joke about his 'huge nose'.

From my own experience, I can see how extreme fatness would act as a barrier. If society tells you that you look 'wrong', if you're too thin or too fat to be considered conventionally 'attractive', you effectively rule yourself out of the dating, career and life rat-race. Not that overweight people don't fall in love and get married – of course they do – but for many, fat is a form of protection, and self-defence. Thin worked the same way for me: at times the world seemed so overwhelming, and the possibilities for success and failure so numerous. Being skeletal, not taking the risk, was my weird way of staying safe.

A final thought on the fat-and-funny theme. In 2012 the comedian Jenny Eclair (as well as having an excellent cake-surname) wrote in the *Radio Times* about her experience of anorexia several decades ago. Her flippant tone disguises what was clearly a very painful time:

> At 19 I went on a diet and I didn't stop dieting for five years. All of a sudden I didn't know how not to be on a diet... I was fascinated by my disappearing flesh. I'd invented a new snack: raw carrots dipped in Marmite. Everyone began to despair. My flatmate tried to cook for me. We fought over her attempt to use butter – a proper physical fight. I threw the butter out the window and then I moved out. It was so much easier to starve alone. (*Radio Times*, August 2012)

Eclair says she hasn't been able to eat chocolate or cake for more than twenty years. Like many women, she still has an 'odd relationship' with food, and still doesn't trust food not to make her fat. Her story surprised me, because she seems so ballsy and full of gusto. I suppose I wouldn't associate such an enfeebling condition as anorexia with such a confident, no-nonsense woman. Then again, it may well have been this sense of not feeling quite right within her own body, which led her to comedy. Being fat doesn't make you automatically funny, but I suspect there is some truth in this observation by the comedian Joan Rivers: 'Why don't beautiful women do comedy? Because they don't have to.'

*

I can't imagine anything more petrifying than stand-up comedy – worse even than a high diving board, or adding butter to toast!

It took many years, but my fear of fat has finally receded. There is something wonderful about facing that fear, and testing it, and conquering it. It's a silly fear which gets weaker every time I enjoy melting Brie on French bread, or a bar of milk chocolate, or pasta drowning in olive oil. My Irish friend was right when she said that double cream thickened up the soup 'something gorgeous' – the taste of fat is unique; the absence of fat in food makes everything taste meagre and somehow flavourless.

The F-word can be scary, and it can be judgemental, but we can't live without it. None of us is immune to the social shudder inherent in the F-word – and at the same time, we are surrounded by sources of delicious food, targeted by food advertisers, and encouraged to treat ourselves. It's hard to find a balance in a world which is so fearful and obsessed with fat – which demonises the shape of fat, the hint or dimple or roll of excess flesh, especially on women. It's no wonder many of us get caught up in the cycle of diet or excess, bingeing or self-denial, fat or thin, all or nothing. Probably the best we can do is to remember the old saying: all things in moderation and moderation in all things.

Chapter 3

THE MINISTRY OF DIETS

Do you recognise any of these rules?

1. If you eat something and no one sees you eat it, it has no calories.
2. If you drink a Diet Coke with a chocolate bar, the calories in the chocolate are cancelled out by the Diet Coke.
3. When you eat with someone else, calories don't count if you don't eat more than they do.
4. Foods used for medicinal purposes NEVER count, such as hot chocolate, brandy, toast and Sara Lee Cheesecake.
5. If you fatten up everyone else around you, then you look thinner.
6. Cinema-related foods do not have calories because they are part of the entertainment package and not part of one's personal fuel. Examples: Popcorn, M&Ms, Wine Gums, Maltesers, Skittles.

7. Broken biscuits contain no calories. The process of breaking causes calorie leakage.
8. Things licked while cooking have no calories if you are in the process of preparing something. You are merely tasting.
9. Anything consumed while standing has no calories. This is due to gravity and the density of the caloric mass.
10. Anything consumed from someone else's plate has no calories since the calories rightfully belong to the other person and will cling to his/her plate. (We ALL know how calories like to cling!)

OK, those are silly rules found on the Internet, but you know the principles. Among my friends, other calories-which-don't-count examples include: 'It doesn't count if it's half, it's tiny or if you're having a green tea after', 'It doesn't count if it's Christmas, Easter, your birthday or someone else's' and 'It doesn't count if it's one of your five a day.' I particularly loved this one: 'It doesn't count if you're going to the gym, been to the gym or are wearing gym gear.'

Maybe we use humour to disguise the fact that, basically, dieting is a depressing business. And futile. The average diet does not work. An estimated 90 per cent of people who lose weight by dieting will regain it within two years. Diets are not only a multibillion dollar industry, they're also something of an occupational obsession: in the past ten years it's estimated that around 70 per cent of the adult female population and 30 per cent of adult males have been on one. Hence the joke: there are two types of women, those who are watching their weight and those who pretend not to be.

It's a Monday-morning institution among my female colleagues, updating who's following which diet from the weekend's magazines, what they are and are not allowed to eat, how much weight they're planning to lose and how quickly, if anyone has ever tried it before, and potential side-effects (e.g. flatulence,

THE MINISTRY OF THIN

sudden fainting, loss of peripheral vision etc.). It's all quite light-hearted. The question, 'What are you on?' is routine and doesn't mean drugs – it means are you on the Paleo Caveman Diet, Atkins, Clean and Lean, liquid-only, whatever.

Like second marriages, diets represent the triumph of hope over experience. No matter how many times dieters try and fail to lose weight permanently, it seems they're always ready to try again. This time, they tell themselves, will be different. But the chances are it won't be.

Unfortunately, going on a diet is not like giving up smoking, where it's been shown that the more attempts you make, the more likely you are to succeed in quitting completely. Although diets often produce results in the short-term, very few dieters maintain their weight loss. Worse, most end up heavier than they were before they started trying to get thin. Here's why diets don't work:

- **Diets are punishing:** It's hard to be hungry all the time, and most people don't like punishing themselves. Diets rely on willpower, long-term determination, and constant self-surveillance. It's easier to treat yourself than it is to deny yourself.
- **Diets make you feel deprived:** They make you hungry and create cravings for the foods you must avoid. It's human nature to want what you can't have. On top of the craving for sugar, fat or carbs is the feeling of deprivation – everyone else is enjoying something you can't have.
- **Diets are tedious:** Maybe you get bored with the rigid eating plan and break the rules. Then you tell yourself you've 'blown it'; this creates a self-fulfilling prophecy, where a small failure leads to a total collapse. You've broken the diets rules so you might as well inhale the rest of the Quality Street selection box.
- **Failure begets failure:** People go from diet to diet, hoping to find the magic one – but it doesn't exist. And since the body doesn't

want to starve, it responds to restrictive diets by slowing your metabolism which makes it harder to lose weight, leading to a cycle of overeating, bingeing, and yo-yo dieting.

- **Diets fail to address the emotional aspect of food:** Many of us over-eat (or under-eat) as a way of coping with, or avoiding, deeper issues. Obviously, food is a rubbish way of dealing with psychological problems.

- **Diets don't change core habits:** The only effective way to lose weight and keep it off is by making permanent changes: to lifestyle, to eating and exercise. Diets are basically short-term – they help you reach your goal weight, but they don't teach you how to stay slim.

In fact, although I have proved myself to be a highly proficient dieter, I don't know much about actual diets. I have never followed The South Beach, Atkins or Dukan: their rules seem so tedious and complicated – I have tried reading those books and got bored after the first chapter. By contrast, the rules of anorexia were simple: eat less, burn more. You can always cut what you're eating in half; you can always increase the amount you're exercising. It's shocking to think of now, but maybe it was this simplicity which appealed to me.

When I talk to people who are trying to lose weight, there seems to be a lot of denial going on. Often it's their genes or their childhood which is to blame for weight, or their stressful job which forces them to eat junk food, or they have no time to exercise. Really these are just excuses to avoid the fundamental truth – if you're overweight you're almost certainly eating too much. It really is that straightforward. A nutritionist I know puts it another way: 'There is no fat person who wouldn't get thin by being locked in a room without food.' It's a basic energy equation: eat less, move more.

But that's kind of tedious – and hard too. How much more exciting to embark on new ways to get thin, from drip-dieting to compulsive porridge-eating, to acupuncture and hypnosis, to food-combining or intermittent fasting, magic powders, pills, even electrode workout machines.

Do you remember that advertisement some years ago, with the lady reclining on the sofa in her bikini with electrode pads attached to her stomach, calmly watching television while she got thin? Did anyone ever lose weight with Electrical Muscle Stimulation, I wonder? There is plenty of hilarity and scepticism about this online – at The Straight Dope Website (Fighting Ignorance Since 1973) a poster called Jayjay comments: 'Honestly... I mean, I'm lazy and fat and all, but at least I don't try to pretend that getting an electrical jolt is the equivalent of exercise.'

I liked the carefully worded Wikipedia entry for Electrical Muscle Stimulation: 'EMS devices cause a calorie burning that is marginal at best: calories are burnt in significant amount only when most of the body is involved in physical exercise... However, some authors imply that EMS can lead to exercise, since a person toning his/her muscles with electrical stimulation is more likely afterwards to participate in sporting activities as the body is ready, fit, willing and able to take on physical activity.'

One can't help but notice that the bodies used to advertise these abdominal toning belts are already very slim (for women) or sculpted (for men).

Most miracle weight-loss products are harmless, or ineffective, but sometimes the desire to get thin can have more dangerous consequences. Back in the mid-1990s the diet drug Fenphen was prescribed to obese Americans until it was found that it could cause fatal heart-valve problems in up to a third of cases. Other commonly abused diet drugs, including Ritalin and Reductil, are a powerful combination of amphetamine and appetite suppressant. They can be highly addictive, and have side effects including insomnia, mood swings, chest pains, palpitations, nausea, headaches, dizziness, anxiety, hallucinations and high blood pressure. Fat binders (such as Xenical and Alli) are even more unpleasant: they work by binding to the fat in food and transporting it out via the bowels, before it can be ingested. The diet drug Qsymia has recently been approved in the US, and claims to help patients lose 10 per cent of their body weight in a year. Obviously none of these slimming 'aids' are healthy or long-term remedies for an unhealthy diet or lifestyle.

I've never tried slimming drugs, but I do know that recreational drugs do funny things to your appetite. Smoking marijuana gives you the most enormous munchies, usually around 2 a.m., when only a greasy kebab, or chips and cheese, will do. Amphetamines ('speed') make you want to dance all night, and often not feel hungry for days. No wonder it used to be taken by dancers, models and other women to stay slim.

Alcohol too has an effect: the most overweight regions of the UK, in the East Midlands and the North, also have problematic levels of binge-drinking. And booze makes you fat: like my friend D says, when he gets a paunch he knows he has to stop drinking beer. Most diets ban alcohol, or only allow it in tiny quantities – 'your evening treat, one small glass of red wine'. (As if!)

When I was anorexic, I never gave up alcohol completely, although I was socialising less and therefore drinking less. Somehow the liquid calories in alcohol weren't as threatening as the calories in food – and I was so light that I'd get tipsy from a few sips of wine. In recent years there have been health concerns about 'drunkorexia', another one of the invented 'exias' to describe an addiction or bad habit – tanning, shopping, dieting etc. Drunkorexia involves 'saving' your calories for binge-drinking. Predominantly young women, drunkorexics starve themselves by day in order to drink themselves silly at night. One blogger commented: *I skip lunch and dinner at weekends in order to save my calories for beer and cocktails LOL. Is there also a 'I'mgoing outforabigmealtonightarexic'?*

*

We diet because we want to change, but where does our desire for change come from? Maybe it's a human instinct to want to improve ourselves; to dream of reinvention by way of the latest food or workout regime, and regular body brushing. We make pledges, promises and New Year's Resolutions. I've probably read more self-help books than I've had hot dinners – I'm a big fan of *Feel the Fear and Do It Anyway* and *The Power of Now*. Among my female friends, we love affirmations and Post-it notes on mirrors and positive mantras. Similarly, men seem to enjoy buying new equipment, whether it's a rowing machine or an elliptical cross-trainer, even if they never use them. We all like the idea of a fresh start.

So it makes sense that we love a new diet. Rather than eating less and running more – how *boring* – we learn intricate rules about zones and blood groups and 'eating right for your type'. We use smaller plates, or we only eat foods of certain colours, or we avoid carbs after 6 p.m. My friend R is currently trying to eat only with her left hand (she's right-handed). It's supposed to slow her down, make her more 'mindful' of her eating, and encourage her to stop when she's full, but she says she's just getting really ambidextrous.

The Atkins Nutritional Approach seemed quite strict when it first appeared, but it's nothing compared to the latest batch of extreme diets. Originally conceived by Robert Atkins in 1972, the revamped Atkins Diet gained widespread popularity in 2003, and in 2004 at the height of its popularity it was estimated that more than 10 per cent of adults in America were on the diet.

The premise for both the Atkins and Dukan diets is simple: protein is good, carbs are bad. They're based on similar lines: no calorie counting, unlimited amounts of meat and a lot of eggs. (As a strict vegetarian with unresolved issues around unfertilised baby chicks, both Atkins and Dukan make me feel a bit queasy.) As well as being low-carb, Dukan is also low-fat, and starts with a short, sharp 'attack' phase, in which nothing but protein is consumed. After a week or so, you alternate protein days with protein and green vegetable days. Once you reach your ideal weight, you can eat anything you want twice a week; but you must continue with protein-only days once a week for the rest of your life.

How can any diet seriously ban fruit and vegetables, ever, and claim to be healthy or balanced? Initially, of course, these carb-free regimes work. Weight-loss occurs quite quickly because the body slips into ketosis mode, and starts to metabolise faster. Unfortunately ketosis also gives you unholy halitosis. A colleague of mine on Atkins suffered constipation, felt dehydrated all the time, and craved fresh fruit. There are many other serious health risks associated with high-protein diets, including loss of bone density from lack of calcium and excessive acidity in the body, and an increased risk of cancer from high meat intake, colon cancer in particular. Carbohydrates are happy foods, boosting serotonin in the brain, so low-carb diets can induce a low mood. There's also the basic fact that these diets are massively lacking in vital fibre, vitamins and minerals. How is this sustainable over a lifetime?

If demonising entire food groups (such as carbs) causes nutritional deficiencies, is it healthier to eat less across the board? Calorie restriction, intermittent fasting and 'alternate-day-diets' have become popular in recent years. Restricting your calories sounds quite radical, as does anything involving the word 'fasting', but it's arguably the most sensible solution when you consider that the majority of us require less energy, to do less movement, than more active, pre-digital, pre-convenience-age generations.

Calorie restriction (CR) is based on the theory that the less you eat, the longer you'll live. Scientific studies have shown that mice and monkeys who are fed very little survive around 50 per cent longer, although it's not clear why this should be, or whether the results are directly applicable to human beings. The aim in CR is to keep the BMI at around 18 (which is just in the underweight range) by eating around 25 per cent less than the daily recommended intake – e.g. daily intake of around 1,500 calories for women, instead of the average recommended UK intake of 2,000.

Of course, calorie restriction sets off alarm bells: it sounds too close to anorexia. (That's probably why CR makes sense to me: it's strict and simple; the rules are clear.) But in fact, carried out systematically, CR is demonstrably healthier than the rapid weight losses and gains of yo-yo dieting – it's a lifestyle change, not a short-term quick-fix. Within the reduced calorie system of CR, nothing is banned; in fact calories need to contain as many nutrients as possible to avoid malnutrition. So CR means a diet containing lots of fruit and vegetables, lean protein and healthy fats. It discourages the consumption of 'empty' calories in sugar, alcohol and junk food. Eating slightly less, but eating healthily, surely makes more sense than gorging on meat and cutting out carbs, or replacing meals with milkshakes. It also avoids the excessive stress which we cause to our bodies when we consume too much and then exercise furiously to burn it off.

The Alternate Day Diet (ADD) is a variation on the theme of calorie restriction. Also known as the DODO diet (day on, day off), ADD works on the principles of 'up' days and 'down' days: on an 'up' day you consume whatever you want (within reason) and on a 'down' day you consume only 500 calories. In theory, the sharp, intermittent reduction in calories makes the body switch on a gene called SIRT1, sometimes called the 'skinny gene', which in turns reduces the amount of fat stored by the body. Unlike CR, which encourages steady, long-term calorie reduction, there is something bingey about ADD, with the hunger of 'fasting' days likely to trigger overeating on 'feasting' days.

So is this a safe way to diet? After all, there is no conclusive health evidence for our accepted 'three meals a day' human habit; it may be that gentle ADD, whereby dieters alternate more treaty days with lighter days, or only restrict their intake a few days a week, is harmless. Yes and no. Alternate day dieting tends to encourage all-or-nothing eating habits, with dieters plotting how best to spread their meagre 500 calories across the down days; and splurging on forbidden high-calorie foods in between. And in its strictest form, ADD can have a detrimental effect on mood and happiness – with 'up' days feeling very 'up' and 'down' days feeling very 'down'.

They may sound radical, but Calorie Restriction and Alternate Day Dieting are nothing compared to the Drip Diet, a liquid-only regime popular with celebrities and brides-to-be who want to lose a lot of weight fast. On this bizarre programme they cut their food intake to 500 calories a day, then go into a clinic every morning and have nutrients fed to them via a drip. (To put that in context, Belsen concentration camp inmates were on starvation rations of somewhere between 600 and 800 calories a day.) The IV drip basically sustains them while they starve their bodies of food. In *Grazia* magazine, one Hollywood publicist said, 'I've had a client who survived on a no-solid-food cleanse for three weeks. She had a drip every morning and managed to lose her goal of 15 pounds, in order to fit into the size zero Oscar dress.'

Or there's the Ketogenic Enteral Nutrition or KEN diet, where a small feeding tube is inserted into the nose, depositing fat, protein and water in the stomach, while simultaneously suppressing the appetite. Apparently patients can expect to lose up to 20 lb in ten days.

If you don't like the idea of an IV drip or a naso-gastric tube, how about injecting pregnancy hormones into yourself? The HCG diet was developed fifty years ago by a British doctor who believed that the HCG hormone – naturally produced by the body during pregnancy – could shift fat by working on the hypothalamus gland which affects metabolism. The HCG diet has become popular in America, even though it has no credible scientific backing and isn't approved by the US Food and Drug Administration. Like Drip dieters, HCG dieters are allowed to eat only 500 calories a day. Then they have a couple of drops of HCG, either injected or on the tongue.

Whether the injection of pregnancy hormones has any effect on weight-loss or not, or is even safe, is kind of beside the point: anyone on 500 calories a day (a few apples and 100 g of protein) will lose masses of weight. Like so many diets, the HCG regime is totally unsustainable in the long-term. Even if you didn't go into manic binge-eating mode, your metabolism would slow right down, and you'd regain weight quickly when you started eating normally.

When I look at diets this insane, I feel comparatively sane. And when I listen to the women around me at work, I feel comparatively healthy. Obviously, working in the media, my colleagues could well be considered more image-conscious than most – but, as I've said before, they talk about diets constantly. They know the caloric content of every food, and indulge in all sorts of dangerous behaviours (including purging) when they have eaten or drunk too much. An entire day's fasting will end with a 5-hour white wine session and a midnight fast food blow-out.

Anorexia is without doubt a serious eating disorder, but there is a hell of a lot of mainstream disordered eating going on out there.

*

Here are just a few of the exchanges which have taken place among my female colleagues:

- 'If you see a calorie pass my lips today, shoot me. Seriously, I was really bad this weekend – this week I'm doing liquid only.'
- 'I've eaten practically this entire packet of Reese's Pieces and I have to wear a bikini in 3 days. I feel sick.'
- 'On Sunday my boyfriend made bacon sandwiches and I ate three rounds...'
- 'You don't need to worry – you're tiny – you literally have no bum, babes!'
- 'So did you get something to eat last night, after the bar?' 'Yeah I got something on the way home, a chicken burger and chilli-cheese fries. Total diet fail...' Cue lots of groaning and laughing all round... 'I know I know! Just don't eat today babes.' 'Yeah, I won't eat all today and tomorrow, it'll be fine.'

Is this the way we all have to be now – deeply anxious over food, constantly watching what we eat, bingeing or starving, or hopelessly trapped on the diet treadmill? Maybe our metabolisms are irrevocably messed up, maybe we've developed such neuroses about food that we'll never know what it's like to eat naturally again. Look at children: if only we could regain that instinctive human response to hunger and appetite. Sometimes it *does* feel like the age of eating innocence is well and truly behind us.

It's easy to despair about all this: imagine a lifetime of dieting stretching ahead. But let's not give up all hope. There's nothing like a bit of humour. I loved Marian Keyes' light-hearted take on diet and deprivation in her blog:

> I was on the Dukan Diet and it plunged me into the most horrific state of mind I've had in a while. Are you familiar with the wretched thing? It's a carb-free – yes, you heard me – CARB-FREE high-protein eating plan which counts as cruel and unusual punishment... I managed to do 10 days but – guess what?! – I put back on 'all' my lost weight as soon as I started eating a 'balanced' diet again. (Balanced diet: 5 parts chocolate cake, 3 parts Percy Pigs, 1 part carrot.)

Like most dieters, eventually, Marian Keyes has accepted that there is no such thing as a miracle diet:

> I am now – sincerely – taking a very long-term attitude to weight-loss... But when the chocolate demons come at me I've discovered it is no good, no good at all, to slowly eat two squares of 70% Green and Black. How I WISH I was that person!

*

Marian's right, strict diets can plunge you into a 'horrific state of mind'. And anorexia is hell. But no one wants to be fat. So what's the solution? Obviously we all know what we should be doing – balancing calories in with calories out – eating fresh, wholesome food and being physically active. It's no surprise that every diet or weight-loss miracle ever invented claims it will be effective *in conjunction with a healthy diet and regular exercise*. We might as well skip the magic powders, expensive injections or the ice-cold baths: it's the healthy eating and exercise that are actually the effective ingredient.

Personally, I'm trying something new. I like the idea of Intuitive Eating. I've been reading about it on the Internet and here are the basic principles:

1.   Reject the diet mentality
2.   Honour your hunger
3.   Challenge the food police
4.   Make peace with food
5.   Respect your fullness
6.   Discover the satisfaction factor
7.   Honour your feelings without using food
8.   Respect your body
9.   Exercise
10. Honour your health

I know it's a bit Californian, but if you can overlook the slightly hippy-sounding notion of 'honouring' your health or feelings, this nutritional philosophy makes a lot of sense. It is based on the premise that eating in response to internal cues of hunger and satiety, while allowing all foods to be a part of the diet, is the way to achieve a healthy weight, rather than calculating calories or fat in foods. The key traits of Intuitive Eating are: unconditional permission to eat, eating for physical rather than emotional reasons, and reliance on internal hunger/satiety cues. It is feeding your body, not your pain/joy/guilt/shame.

This philosophy is more revolutionary than you might think. Imagine if, when you felt hungry, you ate exactly what you wanted – be it a slice of cake or a tin of sardines – regardless of what others were eating, or what you thought you should be eating. You would not get fat from eating the cake – because you wouldn't always want cake – and you would not feel guilty afterwards. You wouldn't be disconnected from your internal hunger cues, and you wouldn't be triggered by external reasons (emotions, 'because it's time', opportunity, or perceived rules of eating).

It's what we're all striving for, isn't it? A more conscious, mindful response to our own appetites. After all, the human body is not preprogrammed to be overweight or underweight: we create these problems by over-eating or under-eating. The diet industry labels foods as either 'good' or bad', marketing hype makes eating either sinful or virtuous, thus causing a sense of deprivation and creating cravings. Intuitive Eating is all about listening to what your body actually needs, rather than using food as a way to numb your feelings, to reward or to punish yourself.

*

I think intuitive eating appeals to me because eating disorders are so unnatural. They mess up simple hunger responses; they destroy what should be our most natural relationship – with our own body. Eating disorders come from a place of profound mistrust. Bulimics and binge-eaters cram in large amounts of 'forbidden' foods; anorexics deny their bodies its most basic human need. Both are forms of self-hatred and self-neglect, you binge or starve and in both cases you become sick and unlovely (which is what you always knew you were, and no less than you deserve).

Intuitive eating seems like a way to reconnect me with myself. Anorexia stems from a terrible need for control, an anxiety that if you let go for a minute, you will spin wildly out of control. I wouldn't withhold food from a friend or a baby like this, so why do I do it to myself? Nor would I ignore feelings of fear or danger; I trust my instincts when it comes to work, personal safety, relationships; so why ignore feelings of hunger? If the strongest message the human body can send – I need food – is repeatedly over-ridden, what can the body rely on?

A few years ago my psychiatrist asked me to go out for dinner with a friend. Eating out in public was something I found very difficult, and she wanted me to do more of it. 'So what will you say?' she asked me. 'You're having a drink at your flat, then I want you to suggest going out to a restaurant.'

I looked at her. 'Well, the party we're going to doesn't kick off until 9ish, so we could get something to eat on the way.' 'Yes', she replied, 'but what will you actually say?'

'I could say, I'm quite peckish – or, have you eaten – shall we get a quick bite before the party?' I felt really unsure of what the correct language is, in this situation. 'I don't know – what would you say?' I asked her. It surprised me, how hard I found it to say those words out loud: 'I'm hungry.'

*

It's still not easy – for me, and for many women – to say those simple words: 'I'm hungry. I need food.' And this, I think, is why intuitive eating appeals to me more than any miracle diet ever could. Diets offer short-term success and long-term failure; an endless cycle of deprivation and guilt. But why shouldn't eating be a pleasure?

All the rule-making and rule-breaking in the world won't fix a bad relationship with food. An intuitive approach to eating doesn't set rules or restrictions – instead it puts you back in touch with yourself. It asks you to respect your own feelings. The more I listen to what my body wants, honour my hunger, and trust my appetite, the happier life becomes.

Chapter 4

THE MINISTRY OF DETOX

'God that smells amazing.' My cousin gazes at my steaming mug of Arabica coffee. 'Let me pour you some,' I say, reaching for the cafetiere. 'No, no, I mustn't. Just hot water is fine,' she says, miserably prodding the slice of lemon. 'Only another two days to go. Just let me smell that coffee again...'

'So what's the deal with this detox – what are you allowed?' I ask, sipping at my caffeine like an addict getting a fix.

'Basically nothing,' she says. 'No wheat and dairy, no red meat, no salt, no tea or coffee, no alcohol, no fizzy drinks, no juice or squash, no refined carbs, no saturated fats, no additives or preservatives. So, no cakes or biscuits, no crisps, no butter or margarine, no mayonnaise or salad dressing, no crisps, no bread or cereal or pasta... The first three days was just steamed vegetables and fish. Now I'm allowed to add rice cakes, stewed fruit and eggs. And I have to drink at least 2 litres of room-temperature water throughout the day, plus dandelion tea and cleansing apple vinegar.'

'But you must feel totally amazing, right?' I ask, sympathetically.

'I feel like shit!' she practically sobs. 'Seriously, look at me – my skin is having some kind of breakout and I'm permanently on the verge of fainting or bursting into tears.' I have to admit, she does look pretty awful. 'I'm ingesting vast quantities of milk thistle complex, psyllium husks and spirulina powder. Plus I can't sleep because I'm so bloody hungry.' She gets a desperate look in her eyes, grabs a packet of Marlboro Lights from her handbag and marches to the balcony. 'I may not be allowed to eat or drink, but I bloody need to smoke.'

So much for detoxing.

*

When I quizzed her more closely, my cousin was vague on precisely what she was detoxing. It was something to do with stimulating her liver, eliminating toxins and allergens, boosting her energy levels, rebalancing herself. However, she admitted that she'd never felt more hungry and tired, and was having hallucinations about chocolate digestive biscuits. So why do we do it?

Among the many 'healthy' obsessions in modern life, surely 'detoxing' is one of the craziest. While evidence of global warming accumulates, and the icebergs melt, while we drive and fly and pollute this fragile planet like never before, we're also paranoid about hygiene, cleanliness and purity. We pay a premium for Fair Trade products and feel better in ourselves for these charitable acts, while plundering the world's natural resources with our relentless hunger for stuff, for travel, for oil, gas, electricity. We recycle our rubbish with painstaking care (my boyfriend has five different bins in his kitchen!) and yet our levels of waste are astonishing. Almost half the world's food is thrown away: we produce more than enough to feed everyone, yet 1 in 8 people on the planet still go hungry.

We scour our bathrooms and kitchens, we wash our clothes and our bodies as if the plague was at the door, we sip volcano, glacier or spring water while a billion people worldwide have no water at all and 3,000 children die each day from diseases caught through drinking tainted supplies. We worry about pollution and yet some of us even pay to have poison injected into our faces, and silicone into our lips and breasts. We panic about the safety of our young children, imagining they're better off indoors with their laptops, smartphones and social networks. We embrace new diets and join gyms and pay over the odds for organic produce, meanwhile our food is more processed, laden with sugar, salt and artificial preservatives than ever before, and the average person's weight is steadily rising. We eat while rushing down the street, watching TV, or on the phone, we wrap our food in plastic which may or may not be carcinogenic (depending on which scare-stories you believe).

These days anything hand-made, farm-sourced or home-spun is automatically superior to any of that store-bought rubbish, right? From artisan chocolate to biodynamic wine, those who can afford it can feel sophisticated, healthy... and just a little bit smug. But we have little cause for smugness while we're dumping garbage and hazardous waste in third-world and developing countries, and polluting their environments with our chemical factories and rapacious demand for trees and water and oil.

So how can we live more 'sustainably', without the complacent connotations attached to that word? We've become addicted to consumerism, it seems. These days you will struggle to get a plumber to look at a broken washing machine or fridge: most will advise you to buy a new one if it's more than a year old. It seems that everything is disposable; everything is short-term. Recently my best friend was getting stressed about the delay in his iPhone upgrade: 'I should be on iPhone 5 by now! I've had the 4 nearly a year, I feel like a dinosaur,' he said. He's right: our mobiles are outdated in a few months, as are our computers, superseded by the latest technology. All our cassettes and CDs – all our stereos for that matter, our Walkmans, our record players – are basically junk, now that everything is online. Sound-system speakers, VHS players, analogue televisions on eBay cost pennies.

I'm not the only one who feels depressed at the wastefulness; bewildered by the impermanence of it all. A similar confusion applies to food: how we should live, what we should eat. Surely most of us would like to live in a less 'processed' way, yet many of us lurch from one miracle detox to the next super-supplement, endlessly looking for that perfect 'natural' balance. Rationally, we know that the surest way to maintain a healthy weight is to eat when we're hungry and stop when we're full; enjoy treats in moderation and stay active. But moderation isn't easy to achieve: instead we go for broke, bingeing on calories and then retreating to the misery of a strict detox.

One of the latest fads is Intermittent Fasting – also known as the 5:2 diet. The idea is that fasting for two non-consecutive days each week (and not on the other five days) can yield terrific benefits; swift, sustainable weight loss without the dreary challenge of calorie control. Apparently periodic fasting not only delivers weight loss, but also cuts your risk of developing cancer and heart disease, boosts energy, mood and brain power, and halts the ageing process… (Just imagine your wonderful mood on those two non-food days.)

Even working out what is considered 'healthy' can be a minefield, let alone actually sticking to it. I'm a fairly well-informed consumer, but I still feel dazed and confused about the cacophony of debate raging about our food: is soya good for you, or has it been linked to breast cancer? Is milk good for your bones, or are cows really being pumped full of artificial hormones?

And what about oily fish – which ones contain dangerous levels of mercury? Wheat and dairy: why so many intolerances these days? Are carbohydrates really the enemy, or a powerful source of energy? What about the Alkaline Diet: why are starchy grains, pasta, wheat and beans, all dairy products, meat and fish classed as 'acid forming'? What does this even mean – are they bad for us? Who invents this stuff; where is the scientific evidence?

Frankly I can't figure out half the ingredients in apparently healthy foods. For example, the mango, papaya and passion fruit yogurt I've just eaten for breakfast. It is labelled 'no preservatives' and yet it contains modified tapioca starch, thickener (guar gum), aspartame, emulsifiers and 'a source of phenylalanine'. What are these sinister-sounding chemicals, and why are they necessary? Some nutritionists say we should avoid eating anything where we can't identify all the substances listed on the label, but of course it's not that simple.

We've known about the health benefits of fresh, unprocessed food for years. But look at the way things have changed recently: beauty and fitness and food are a focus of near-obsession for many magazines, websites and TV programmes. It's like we've been taken in by this colossal detox-scam: we've agreed that we are surrounded by invisible 'toxins' and in need of purification, despite scientific evidence to the contrary. The nutritionist Ian Marber commented on Twitter the other day: 'You don't need to try to "detox" any more than you need to try to breathe. It happens anyway.' And he's right: apart from the liver, which clearly benefits from alcohol-free regeneration, the rest of our organs don't actually need detoxification.

Only a few decades ago perfectly healthy people would have looked at you blankly if you'd suggested 'going on a detox'. Terms such as low-carbing, clean eating, or juicing had not been invented, and the notion of 'flushing out toxins' would have been incomprehensible. Previous generations ate well, with a good balance of food groups, without worrying about Glycaemic Index, slow-release carbs, or antioxidants.

Remember those comments from the *Sydney Morning Herald*? 'The ability to select and consume biodynamic, macrobiotic, locally sourced and fully organic food is surely the greatest middle-class indulgence of our time.' Think of the relish with which we use those terms: sustainable, seasonal, free-range, farm-reared, ethically sourced. We pay a premium for our probiotics and our antioxidants, we're suckers for a detox diet, but do we really know what we're paying for? How would you actually define 'superfood'? Of course you've heard the marketing spiel: superfoods are nutritional 'powerhouses' packed with antioxidants, polyphenols, vitamins and minerals, they are wonder foods, miracle workers. However, the term 'superfood' is rarely used by dieticians or nutritional scientists, many of whom dispute that particular foodstuffs have any of the so-called 'super' health benefits.

In fact, there is no independent definition of 'superfood'. It is not a term used by nutritional science or dieticians, nor is there any legal consensus as to what constitutes a 'superfood'. Rather it's an unscientific marketing term used to describe foods which are free of artificial ingredients, additives or contaminants, and high in nutrients or phytochemicals. This is a pretty accurate definition of most fruit and vegetables. Currently fashionable superfoods include blueberries (or goji berries, or acai berries), broccoli, spinach, pumpkin and tomatoes – and we pay a premium for them. Commoner plant foods such as apples, carrots and potatoes are super-healthy too, but are rarely touted as 'super'.

The marketing of trends such as 'superfoods' is all-important. Whether it's the anti-ageing benefits of oily fish, or the purity of organic milk, even the savviest consumer will find it hard not to be influenced to some degree. Recently a leaflet on my doormat offered me 'a range of superfighting antioxidants for anti-ageing, digestion and proven health benefits, with the purest natural ingredients sourced from all over the world. Seaweed from the Adriatic, Krill from the Antarctic, and Black Rice Bran from China.' And superfoods aren't the only modern miracle we're being peddled – what about the supplements we're encouraged to wash down with our morning wheatgrass shot? Some days, after my cocktail of essential fish oil, calcium, vitamins C and D, zinc, magnesium and evening primrose oil, I feel like I'm rattling.

Exotic, superfighting, and somehow wild! The element of wildness appeals to many of us – we go mad for the Paleo 'Caveman' diet, we like the idea of foraging for nuts and berries, eating raw, eating clean. We believe that fungi, squirrel, wood sorrel or whatever, will cleanse and purify us, as if more expensive nutrition will make us into better people. By getting closer to nature we feel purer, wilder – and for some of us, thinner. It was clear in Liz Hurley's comments about 'shop-bought cakes' that now, more than ever before, there is a moral dimension to our food tastes and behaviour. It's not just what we eat, it's who we are.

I was reminded of the lifestyle prominence we've given to food recently, when I was selling my flat. After measuring up and taking photographs, the estate agent said: 'Don't forget, the smell of baking bread and roasting coffee is the way to attract buyers!' He was half-joking, but he had a point. People who bake their own loaves or grind their own coffee beans tend to be of a certain type; and when you're selling a flat you're selling a lifestyle.

*

Away from the shops, the general obsession with food and eating persists. At home, relaxing with the Sunday papers, you're bombarded with food supplements, recipes, restaurant reviews. Almost every interview with a female celebrity opens with a description of their weight or body shape, how young/old they look ('fresh-faced and make-up free, it's hard to believe she's in her early forties') and then of course the reference to the meal/ snack the interviewer and actress/musician/model will share. In her 'Lunch Date' feature for *Glamour* magazine, journalist Celia Walden actually lists the dishes beside the interview, so we can work out the caloric damage.

If you try to write an article about a female celeb without mentioning their weight or the contents of their plate, it will be sent back by your editor: I know, I've tried it. Age, shape and food are part of setting the scene – but only for women. The less women eat, especially high-profile women, the more they claim to eat. It used to be that women expressed their femininity by watching their figures, with delicate, bird-like nibbling at table. We've now come full-circle in the food and women situation, so that the thinnest celebs pretend to eat masses!

Here is the opening of a recent *Sunday Times* interview with a British model: 'Jourdan Dunn is so extraordinarily gorgeous that as she sashays through the restaurant in Chelsea where we are meeting for lunch, I almost have to rub my eyes just to make sure I'm seeing her straight. With her exquisitely elongated limbs, a thick curtain of dark hair and mesmerizingly feline eyes, I want to shrink her and put her in my pocket, just to look at when the world seems grey and ugly... Still, there's no phone throwing or diva tantrums here. Tucking into a huge plate of roast lamb with potatoes and gravy, Dunn is sweet and unassuming...'

Or this, from *The Sun*'s *Fabulous* magazine: 'Caroline polishes off her fish-finger sandwich and chips, practically licking the plate clean. A female celebrity who actually enjoys her food – how novel.' (Would they comment on a male celebrity finishing his lunch?)

An actress school-friend of mine who isn't Hollywood-famous but has been in several successful films recognises the interview-eating format here. She tells me:

If I've got a part coming up I have to lose weight – that's part of the look. I'm not naturally thin so I have to really starve myself, it's just what you do. But when you're doing publicity you have to order something hearty like a full English breakfast – interviewers always notice. I make up for it by skipping dinner the night before.

The point for these actresses, models or celebrity interviewees is to look like a superwoman; to appear naturally slim and healthy without even trying that hard – unlike normal women who struggle with their weight. Of course it's not our actual job to look slim and beautiful; we don't have personal trainers or chefs to hone our bodies and our diets. But those superbodies still make us feel inadequate, especially when they make it seem effortless.

A particularly nauseating example of 'oh, I eat everything, me' comes from our farmer friend, Elizabeth Hurley. You may recall the infamous six-raisins interview back in 2006, to launch her beachwear range, where Hurley revealed that she ate just one meal and precisely six raisins a day, in order to fit into her signature skin-tight white jeans. But she recently confided to *Zest* magazine how much more she eats than her partner, the cricketer Shane Warne: 'Shane is very disciplined when he has to be but, bizarrely, I eat at least three times more than him because I'm far greedier and think about food all day long. He's naturally very athletic because he's been a professional sportsman for over twenty years. He keeps threatening to make me run with him, but I've resisted so far!'

Also in the weekend magazines are the quick-fire 'what do you eat' interrogations. My sisters and I are hooked on the *Sunday*

Telegraph's 'My Day on a Plate' feature, in which a public figure pretends to submit everything they've consumed in a single day to the scrutiny of a dietician. This is usually a soap star, actress or former athlete, and they trot out the same 'balanced' diet every week, with a 'naughty treat' thrown in to make it seem more realistic.

A typical breakfast will be egg-white omelette with wholemeal toast (as if anyone has time in the morning), lunch is a large salade niçoise, a handful of nuts for an afternoon snack on the go, and grilled chicken with loads of veggies for dinner, with one glass of wine (ha). If this was really all they ate they'd be ravenous, but the dietician commends them for their slow-release carbs and balanced approach to food – and us readers end up feeling greedy, wobbly and unbalanced as a result.

Here is an example, a singer in a girl-band, from August 2012:

6.30 a.m. It's another early start with my three-month-old baby. Have a glass of orange juice before getting ready for a magazine photo-shoot... 7 a.m. Get picked up. Wake up properly with a cup of tea with a dash of soya milk at the studio, and some granola with soya yogurt, then into hair and make-up. 11 a.m. Mid-morning banana. I prefer snacking on fruit and vegetables to sweets. A packet of crisps is as naughty as it gets. 1 p.m. We get to order in food while we're on set. I love chicken noodle soup or, if it's really hot weather, just a cold ham salad. 4 p.m. With six or seven outfit changes to get through we won't finish until 6 p.m., so I snack on cashew nuts for energy. 7 p.m. My husband does most of the cooking so I nibble on olives while he cooks wholewheat pasta with grilled salmon and broccoli splashed with soy sauce. I love my greens. Afterwards, just a cup of tea.

And here is the dietician's verdict:

If she were trying out for the most virtuous eater of the year, she'd surely be in the top three. She must be one of those very lucky people who doesn't get a rush of anticipation at the sight of cakes, doughnuts or chocolate. Her diet is near perfect and ticks pretty much all the healthy-eating boxes.

＊

'You know that stuff solidifies inside you?' I stare at my big sister. One minute I'm cracking open a lovely cold can of Diet Coke, next thing she's telling me that this afternoon pick-me-up is putting me in mortal danger... 'Apparently the aspartame turns to formaldehyde, or something – I read about it online.'

She's not the only one. In recent years, aspartame has been linked with health risks including multiple sclerosis, systemic lupus, methanol toxicity, blindness, spasms, shooting pains, brain seizures, headaches, depression, anxiety, memory loss, birth defects and even death.

Oh great. So now my Diet Coke is going to kill me. As far as I can see, it's the only thing I love which is truly calorie-free. And now it's the devil's own drug. Would your diet tick all the healthy-eating boxes?

Why do I worry about drinking a Diet Coke once in a while? I could be hooked on heroin, crack cocaine, or alcohol, I could still be smoking for goodness' sake! Years ago I weaned myself off full-fat (sugary) Coke for the calorie-free version – and now even that is bad for me. Is nothing pleasurable allowed any more? A chemical in Coke's caramel colouring was at the centre of a cancer link in the United States. Coca-Cola has recently switched to a new manufacturing process in America to bring down the level of the suspect chemical, 4-methylimidazole (4-MI).

There is something fearful about the way we live. A recent issue of *Good Housekeeping* magazine led with a health feature in which type 2 diabetes was described as 'The Silent Epidemic'. The magazine went on to list the following warning signs: 'Do you eat on the run? Do you have difficulty sleeping? Do you wake up needing a pee? If you recognise any of these signs, you may be at risk.' Surely we could all answer yes, at times, to all these signs.

In the same issue, another article opened: 'Did you know, your handbag is home to more bugs than the average toilet handle...' Overleaf was a sinister Corsodyl mouthwash advertisement: 'Many people think bleeding gums are normal. They're not.' It goes on to warn that spitting blood when you brush your teeth could be an early sign of gum disease, and that 79 per cent of those over thirty-five have gum disease, which leads to more teeth falling out than tooth decay. I know they're probably right, but they don't half make you feel alarmed.

The most preposterous claim I've encountered recently is that of 'toxic paper'. Apparently the Swedish government is concerned that credit card receipts and restaurant bills may increase the risk of cancer. They are proposing a ban on the thermal paper these receipts are printed on because it contains cancer research's latest bugbear: bisphenol A (BPA). Forget the scare stories about plastic packaging contaminating our food, or mobile phone radiation zapping our brains, now we can get cancer from inhaling our receipts. But, reading the research, it's hard not to feel alarmed. BPA is one of the most widely manufactured chemicals, a synthetic oestrogen that can disrupt hormones. It was banned in baby bottles in the EU. There's little evidence as to how much exposure you might get from handling receipts and tickets, but the Swedish Chemicals Agency said that banning BPA would be a move towards a 'toxin-free environment'. (As a cyclist, it often occurs to me: if we're genuinely concerned about toxins, we could start with the black stuff pouring out of the exhaust pipes of cars, buses and lorries. It may be lead-free these days, but it's still deeply unpleasant to cycle through.)

Is it any wonder we're so terrified of germs, toxins, oxidants? The twenty-first century has been called the digital age, but in many ways it's also the age of fear. We no longer allow our children to play in the street, or talk to strangers; we worry about invisible radiation and pollution; and we fuss endlessly about the source of food – the hidden horse-meat revelations are reaching panic-proportions as I write.

And then there is the water in our taps. Because food isn't our only health-worry: water is another source of guilt and anxiety. From the 1990s bottled water has been strategically presented to appeal to consumers, convincing them of the quality, necessity and enjoyment of something they can get from their taps. Despite the fact that over 780 million people still use unsafe drinking water (WHO/UNICEF); despite the fact that we're incredibly fortunate in the developed world to have safe water on tap, still we've been brainwashed by the talk of seven-step filtration, volcanic rocks and pure mountain springs. The fact is that bottling and transporting water for Americans alone uses up 912 million gallons of oil per year. Anti-Water Bottle campaigns here and in the US are fighting to change consumption habits, and there are signs that we may finally be seeing sense. These days it's perfectly acceptable – in a responsible, green way – to order a jug of 'tap' rather than bottled water. It's almost cool.

The Times' restaurant critic Giles Coren has strong opinions on the water issue: 'Mineral water is a preposterous vanity... While half the world dies of thirst or puts up with water you wouldn't piss in, or already have, we have invested years and years, and vast amounts of money, into an ingenious system which cleanses water of all the nasties that most other humans and animals have always had to put up with, and delivers it, dirt-cheap, to our homes and workplaces in pipes, which we can access at a tap... And yet last year we bought three billion litres of bottled water. 3,000,000,000 litres!'

One of my friends in his thirties refuses to drink water from the tap. He lugs crates of Evian water back from the supermarket each week, and even uses it when brushing his teeth. Perfectly rational in other ways, he gets this dark, haunted look when he tells me about the desalination plants, the chemical treatment of water in our sewers – and how many times each drop of drinking water has passed through the bladders of other Londoners.

This paranoia about water taps into a deep insecurity within us. What are these so-called toxins we imagine pouring out of our taps? I'm not referring here to countries where the water isn't clean – I've experienced the horrible effects while on holiday of drinking *eau non potable* – and yes, brushing one's teeth in dirty water can cause diarrhoea. Of course it's sensible to boil or sterilise this water, to avoid salads and fruit which have been washed in dirty water, even ice cubes. But there are no proven health risks associated with drinking tap water in the UK.

Step forward the great detox racket. Of course stylish water is a nonsense. Vast food and beverage companies have been able to convince us to buy exceptionally expensive water as a status symbol, simple as that. We have been brainwashed into believing that bottles of water, with their slick packaging and fancy names, are sexy. Jennifer Aniston, for example, is the face of Glaceau's Smart Water; other celebrities endorse Vitamin Water, or this or that.

It's weird that water has become a status symbol. I asked my eighteen-year-old cousin what three things she couldn't be without, and she instantly replied, 'iPhone, sunglasses, bottle of water'. (She probably also needs her house-keys and wallet, but those weren't the items she listed.) So what's with the H_2O? Is there a looming drought which only the beautiful people know about? If you think about it, it's quite bizarre to tote water around, as if one can't survive a ten-minute bus ride without hydration. Like the takeaway coffee cup, the handbag or the yoga mat, bottled water is another one of those celebrity props/security blankets. We're used to seeing the beautiful ones leaving the gym, clutching a bottle of water: shorthand for I'm successful, busy, super-active.

Bottled or tap, most of us believe that 2 litres of water is what we should be aiming for. Even the British Dietetic Association recommends we drink 1.8 litres of water – around eight glasses – a day. But this misconception is not supported by research. Reviews of all the scientific literature (2002 and 2008) found no solid scientific evidence that recommended drinking eight glasses of water per day. In another triumph of marketing over common sense, we've become convinced that we need to be constantly waterlogged in order to flush out the toxins.

*

Ah yes, the toxins. Because as well as the organic food, purified water and vigorous exercise, we also need to eliminate hidden poisons. Many of us don't even trust our own bodies to function at the most basic level: shifting unwanted waste products through our digestive system and out the other end. We're fixated on purifying ourselves in a way which makes no sense to older generations. My mother had never heard of exfoliation or body-brushing until my sisters and I started all that nonsense. She washes with soap and warm water, moisturises with simple Baby Lotion, and her skin looks young and wrinkle-free for her age.

Compare that to the facial scrubs, loofahs and muslin cloths in my bathroom...

I blame colonic irrigation, which tried to convince us that we were full of nasties which needed pumping out. Surely irrigation is for fields, not human beings! Nonetheless, for a time alternative-health nuts went mad for colonics; journalists wrote articles describing in gruesome detail the hydrotherapy hoses which sluiced out the inner contents of their intestines and rectum. Fortunately, there is no scientific evidence for colon cleansing. The human bowel itself is not dirty, and a healthy digestive system is perfectly able to clear out waste. Colonics can actually cause dangerous infection or bowel damage. What is the earthly point of pumping gallons of water into ourselves when the human body carries more than 100 trillion bacteria?

And do you remember those truly grim foot patches? Although they never caught on, they're still available on the Internet. The theory is that you stick the patches on your feet before bed and they suck the toxins down through the soles of your feet as you sleep. 'Overnight, toxins and body waste will be drawn out into the patch... Through the process of osmosis, the healing properties of the natural ingredients will have been absorbed.'

I never tried them – the images of disgusting blackened patches were enough to put anyone off – but surely we can't really have been so gullible. What are these 'toxins' we imagine floating around inside us; what proof is there that they exist? We have state-of-the-art refrigeration and 'best before' dates, we have more stringent health and safety rules than at any time in history, and much cleaner homes, and yet we still believe that our bodies need purging. I recently bought myself an expensive face cream which promises to fight 'free radicals'. But I've never had any trouble from these so-called free radicals – so why would I want to fight them?

The beauty industry has jumped on the detox bandwagon in a big way, as have peddlers of deodorant, shower gels and other hygiene products. My parents think it's madness the way my brothers, sisters and I shower daily. Personally I need a morning shower and a bedtime bath. And a quick shower after work if I'm going out again in the evening. Or if I've been on the London Underground, or cycling around town. I don't have OCD particularly, I just like feeling fresh. To many of my parents' generation all this washing is simply unnecessary, and wasteful. They're not dirty: they have an all-over wash every morning, and a bath at weekends – whether they need it or not! As children, we had the pre-school Sunday-evening bathtime ritual once a week, often with two or three of us sharing it at the same time.

There is a clear parallel between our fear of invisible toxins and the mania for personal cleanliness: a sense that germs lurk in every corner, a desire to purify ourselves outside as well as in. It makes good sense to supply hand-sanitising gel at the entrance to hospital wards, but these days they're in offices and many homes too. We are fastidious, almost phobic, about natural germs, even though logically we must understand that we're swarming with them. We have entire microbial colonies in our mouths, noses, guts, vaginas, and all over our skin. Again, the cleanliness craze has been a huge marketing opportunity. Since the age of fourteen I have, as instructed by the beauty industry, been exfoliating three times a week with my almond grain and avocado face scrub. It gets rid of dead skin cells apparently (as if they don't fall away naturally). What would happen if I stopped, I wonder – would my face-skin build up and become all dead and unsightly?

It's not such a leap to see our frantic cleansing and scrubbing as the modern equivalent of the medieval hair-shirt. Look at those horrifying chemical peels, where an acidic solution is applied to the skin that causes it to blister and peel off. The new, regenerated skin is apparently smoother and less wrinkled than old skin. You can also opt for laser resurfacing (like a car, or a wall) or dermabrasion, to improve conditions such as acne, sun-pigmentation or wrinkles. Until quite recently, the term 'abrasion' was a bad thing! The actress Jennifer Aniston stays youthful in her forties with regular face peels, and has cheerfully described looking like a 'burn victim' for days afterwards.

OK, the average beauty treatment is less painful than that – but plucking and waxing can be agony. I used to grit my teeth in order not to yelp when I was having underarm laser hair removal. And I have been brought to the verge of tears on more than one occasion by the 'extraction' process during a facial. Seriously, try it.

*

I don't know what we're looking for, with all this purging and scrubbing, the body-brushing and detoxing. It's as if there is something inside of ourselves that we need to scourge. The concept of purity fascinates me: when I was in treatment for anorexia, my psychiatrist and I frequently discussed this. It was clear to us both that my low body weight had less to do with looking 'good' (a common misconception about anorexia) than it had to do with purity and control, and some kind of withdrawal from the messy, chaotic world. Life, and to some extent femininity, *is* curiously uncontrollable – the bloodiness, the curves and the leakage. In my memoir *An Apple a Day*, I recalled the session when my psychiatrist first suggested that anorexia might represent something deeper than just an eating disorder...

I had confessed an element of distaste for flesh and blood femaleness; the voluptuousness of pregnancy; the unpredictability of childbirth and motherhood. He casually observed that in the Middle Ages I might have been a nun: 'an ascetic devoted to denying the demands of the flesh'. I knew instantly what he meant. My private world, my pristine flat, it's controllable, contained and neat. We talked about this – the pain and reward of self-denial, and why it appealed to me.

Dr R had identified something about me that I'd never realised: that the anorexia (even more than thinness) satisfies a yearning for something clean and empty. A part of me fears being womanly, fleshy, excessive: I like to be lithe and compact, I like my tone and muscle. I like to run for miles and feel that I am contained in an athletic body. Being a woman is messy: being a woman involves blood and fat. Anorexia seems very pure and I like that.

In many ways anorexia was like an extreme detox regime: I was addicted to self-denial. The hardest part of recovery wasn't gaining weight: it was giving up renunciation. But it was impossible to have a fully loving relationship when I couldn't allow others in. Sharing the pleasure of food was central to this. When I started eating again my boyfriend and I were able to enjoy special meals: cooking dinner together for our anniversary, or sandwiches in the park, or toast and marmalade in bed at weekends. As anorexia receded, I learned that eating with others creates intimacy and trust. Self-starvation is an intensely isolating experience. Similarly, the process of detox is anti-enjoyment: it makes you wary of everything.

One Sunday morning last year, I asked my boyfriend what my recovery meant to him. He put down his coffee and was silent for a minute: 'I suppose I began to believe that recovery was actually possible. For so long I encouraged you to try new foods, to remind you that I'm here, to reassure you that you'll never get fat. But to be honest Em, I sometimes felt I was wasting my breath. Every time I turned my back you would be secretly swimming or running, dodging meals, losing weight on some insane detox regime…'

I remember how concerned he would get when I mentioned the word 'detox'. Of course there's nothing wrong with having a spell of healthy eating, or taking a break from alcohol, but my concept of detox always went further than that. Fasting is really unnecessary; he was right to be alarmed.

*

During the recent London Fashion Week, I was sent a sample 'nutritious yet delicious' lunchbox from Premier Models. Given the debate around eating disorders and size zeros in the modelling world, I was curious to see what they were feeding their models. Here's the press release which accompanied the lunchbox: 'With raw protein bars, iodine-rich seaweed and power snacks such as almonds, goji berries and pumpkin seeds, this is the perfect handbag-sized snack solution for time-poor health nuts.' Model munchies.

Just as I identified with the self-mortification of those fourteenth-century female mystics, starving and praying in their lonely cells, so I understand the obsession with detoxing. Of course we don't all take it too far; I know that I went way overboard. But probably we can all identify with the sense of moral superiority when we exercise hard, when we buy organic and mix our own sea-salt body scrubs and 'eat clean'. The virtuous glow of not succumbing to the 4 p.m. chocolate craving; the smugness of ordering a salad and a sparkling water.

As a former food-dodger, I think there's more to our modern mania for detox than simply cleansing. Many women – myself included – have used detox regimes as an excuse to avoid food: a seven-day juice fast say, or just fruit until lunch, or no-meat-no-carbs-no-dairy for a month. But this is a profoundly disordered way to eat. Intermittent Fasting, or the Alkaline Diet, or Raw Food, or Protein-Only, it's the same all-or-nothing nonsense by another name. The growing obsession with detoxification is just another manifestation of our warped desire for the perfect diet, the perfect body, the perfect life.

Chapter 5

THE MINISTRY OF GYM

Take your clothes off and stand in front of a large mirror in good light. Let it all hang out and don't look to your partner for reassurance. Tell yourself the ugly truth about your reflection and remember it whenever you are considering skiving a run.

Bracing advice from *Run Fat Bitch Run* by Ruth Field. The book itself has nothing new to say about weight-loss; as we all know it's about exercising more and eating less. But the approach is a combination of cruelty and humour, which I find oddly appealing. The author, who calls herself the Grit Doctor, admits: 'I call myself a fat bitch and laugh my way into my trainers.' And she refuses to make allowances or accept the usual excuses, the commonest being, 'I don't have time to exercise'. We waste so much time and energy finding reasons not to exercise, she argues – in the end you have to just do it.

Most of us are not doing very much at all. According to Baroness Tanni Grey-Thompson, Paralympian and parliamentarian, '80 per cent of women are not doing enough exercise to stay healthy'. We work in sedentary jobs, travel by car, and shop online; interactions with friends are virtual, via Facebook, Twitter and mobile phone, rather than in person. The daily opportunities for physical activity are shrinking. Most of us are literally not burning off the calories we are taking in. Think back to the 1940s or 1950s, when people were working in the fields or in factories, walking to the shops and carrying shopping bags home, cycling to school, sweeping the floors, washing the family laundry by hand. They didn't join gyms because they didn't need to. Today, our lives are arranged for maximum convenience and minimum effort. We really need to move.

I know it's hard. I run three or four mornings a week and it's an effort every single time. I hear my alarm and drag myself out of bed and into my shorts and trainers almost before I'm awake. If I thought about exercising, I would find a reason not to. I try to make the routine as simple as possible: no shower, just put on trainers, brush teeth, inhale a mug of instant coffee and get outside. That's why the Nike slogan is spot-on: *Just do it.*

But it doesn't get any easier. Still, as I'm standing there in my running gear, gulping down the Nescafé, wiring up my iPod, I'd give anything, anything, not to leave the warm flat. And yet I love running (or rather, I love having been for a run); I love being outdoors on freezing winter mornings and on glittering summer dawns; I love being athletic and neat; I love passing other runners by the Regent's Canal and exchanging complicit smiles. More than anything I love standing in the shower, exhausted and invigorated, fresh and clear-headed, making proper coffee and breakfast afterwards. And the feeling which lasts all day, that I've already done the hardest thing I had to...

Because that's the truth: running is hard. And that's why it works. I use running as an example, as it's what works for me, but any intense exercise will do: you're sweating because your heart rate is elevated, because your blood is pumping and your muscles are working hard. When I first hit the pavement I hate it – I feel like the dustman is laughing at me, the bus passengers are staring, all I want to do is turn around and go back indoors. I once read about the 'toxic ten minutes' in *Runner's World*, so I remind myself it's just the first ten minutes, it's toxic for everyone, it will get better. And generally it does. Of course there are days when the whole four or five miles is rubbish: when I'm breathless and I can't get any rhythm going and my feet are leaden. Usually that's when I'm running with a hangover. But there isn't a single morning when I've come back from a run feeling worse than when I left – always better. If nothing else, nothing at all, you've been for a run.

And there are the rare moments, running through Hyde Park, or along the Embankment, when everything falls into place. Rare moments when my legs and arms are working in perfect coordination, when I'm pushing myself hard but not on the verge of collapse, when a great song comes on and I'm Mo Farah, Jess Ennis and Paula Radcliffe rolled into one. Cue 'Eye of the Tiger'!

Yes, music helps: for me it has to be something loud and upbeat, and the cheesier the better – Queen, Beyoncé, Black-Eyed Peas or the theme tune to *Rocky* (anything to block out the sound of my own hyperventilation). And then there are the motivational mantras. When I took up running my best friend would send random texts such as these:

- There is no 'Y' in running. Believe in the run.
- It's what you have left after you give 100 per cent.
- Impossible is nothing.
- Losers let it happen, winners make it happen.
- There is no finish line.

Obviously, he finds them hilarious. But I'm the one who's running!

*

When chatting to colleagues and friends about exercise, you often hear comments like: *You have so much nervous energy*; or – *Oh, you couldn't be fat if you tried*. The implication is that some people are just naturally slim. But scratch the surface of any 'naturally slim' person and I guarantee you will find quite a lot of physical activity, whether that's actual exercise, or simply walking everywhere. So, when I hear people making excuses for being overweight or out of shape, I don't really buy it. Because (a) exercise works; (b) most cyclists and runners are slim; and (c) you don't see fat skeletons. It's not rocket science.

It's hardly surprising that obesity is growing among children. They spend more time in front of televisions, laptops and computer games than they do in the fresh air, often snacking on processed food and sugary drinks. When we were children we walked home from school, changed out of our school uniform and then played in the street. We ran around Camden Town with the other kids, we climbed trees and roller-skated and played hopscotch and French elastic, we had near-misses with cars and buses, we got filthy, we got into endless trouble. Then we went home and ate supper, and that was that. We were constantly covered in bruises and scrapes, but in all that activity no one had a chance to become overweight.

When I go back to Camden now to see my parents, there's simply no after-school activity. We lived out our lives on those streets: the first bike accident, the first kiss or first cigarette, the tree my brother fell out of, the dangerous railway lines we explored. There are still plenty of children in the neighbourhood – working class, middle class – but they're kept safely indoors. The irony of course is that keeping children 'safe' indoors, secure in their bedrooms, is anything but safe. We imagine the outside world is fraught with dangers for our youth, that there's a paedophile on every street corner, but this is far from true. Britain is one of the safest countries in the world – although you wouldn't know it from our levels of fear and suspicion – and the actual risk from strangers is very low. In fact, a terrifying 95 per cent of child sexual abuse is carried out by a perpetrator known to the victim – 60 per cent of abusers actually live in the same house as their victim – a stark reminder that home can be more dangerous than the outside world.

The real risks these days come from the online world: inappropriate contact with predatory adults and so-called grooming are a much greater threat than random abduction. Tragic (but very rare) cases of child kidnapping or murder are widely publicised by the media, fuelling the general climate of panic about 'stranger danger'. Meanwhile, online, children as young as four and five are coming across horrifically adult images, and teenage boys are becoming addicted to the most explicit forms of Internet pornography. In a *Sunday Times* article the journalist Eleanor Mills pointed out: 'These days everything from television to music videos, Instagram to the mania for sexting demonstrates the pervasive pornification of youth culture' (February 2013). She cites research from HealthyMinds.com which found the average age of first exposure to pornographic images is six, and that the largest consumers of Internet pornography are the twelve to seventeen age group.

Additionally, social networks such as Facebook can expose children to cyber-bullying as cruel as anything they might experience in the playground. So our children are not safer when we keep them indoors, wrapped in cotton wool.

Nor are they healthier. My parents always took the view that children are like dogs – they should be outside as much as possible – and I agree. I feel terribly sad when I see overweight youngsters

– not only because they seem so awkward, so encumbered, but because it's such a difficult start in life. More than 80 per cent of overweight children will go on to be overweight adults. A child shouldn't be weighed down with excess bodyweight, or self-hatred, or trying to diet; they should be active and carefree and able to join in.

So, if overweight children become overweight adults, what's the solution? A friend of mine at university had been clinically obese since childhood. Then in our final year, she lost nearly five stone and has kept it off ever since. When I email her now to ask what worked for her, and what changed, she immediately emails back: 'I was eating way too much and I was lazy. I stopped eating junk, I ate less overall, and I started coming to the gym with you guys. It wasn't easy but it was that simple.'

I think she's right, it's not easy but it is simple. Most excuses for not exercising are fairly flimsy when you think about them:

- *I don't exercise because I don't have time*: everyone has 20 minutes a day to run around the park.
- *I don't exercise because I can't afford to join a gym*: going for a run is free.
- *I don't exercise because I'm self-conscious, other people will stare at me*: no one's looking at you. If you jog around the park a few times, no one will notice. Or wait until darkness falls and go running undercover. Or get an exercise DVD and draw the curtains and do it alone. Get sweaty, get out of breath.

Lest I sound evangelical, let me explain: I'm really not a fitness fanatic. I don't lecture friends and family on the joys of exercise or try to persuade them to join me. I am a recent convert to the benefits of exercise. Also, I have to admit that with anorexia, there were many unhealthy aspects to my running. Such as...

- If I didn't run, I felt guilty – I felt that I'd let myself down.
- When I couldn't run for a few days, I became depressed and lethargic – even on holiday.
- I lied about running – I gave it up for 9 months but then started again in secret.
- I always ran alone; I would never share this activity with anyone else.
- The day I gave up smoking I started running.
- Around the same time I also gave up Prozac.

Cross-addicted, ever?

Looked at objectively, there were clear parallels in my addictions to self-starvation and running: the compulsion, the feelings of guilt, the sense of release. There was something very pure about running – no equipment or anyone else involved – just as anorexia is the epitome of purity. The solitariness of running, the fiercely private nature of anorexia. And physically, the two conditions complemented each other – the endorphin-rush I derived from running was perfectly mirrored in the manic, hungry high of anorexia. Both starvation and running lock you into a battle with yourself; both activities alter your brain chemistry. Looking back, I can see that I was subconsciously self-medicating: the serotonin boost I needed from Prozac, I began to get from exercise. And there was a great deal of fear in recovery from anorexia: as I started to gain weight I also stepped up my weekly mileage.

It's only now, in a much healthier place, I can see that exercise had become an addiction. These days I continue to run, but I'm no longer hooked: there is no guilt or secrecy involved. I don't get depressed if I don't have time to exercise. On a winter-sunshine break in Cape Town recently I forgot to pack my trainers so I couldn't run for two whole weeks. Yes, I missed it, but I wasn't anxious about it.

Like most women, I exercise to ensure that I'm not becoming overweight, lazy or (god forbid) relaxed. And like most of us, I feel tempted to skip the exercise routine, and pleased with myself when I don't. But I don't think there's anything inherently superior about the super-fit; in fact I find the whole gym culture intensely irritating. I spent my entire school-career avoiding team sports: I was always picked last for netball and rounders, and totally rubbish at lacrosse. I was active but never 'sporty'.

I'm still not 'sporty', and running takes a hell of an effort. With the rare exception, I think most people have to undergo this mental battle with themselves every time they drag their reluctant bones to the swimming pool, the park or the gym. As well as the physical effort of exercise, it requires a certain mental discipline. At the end of a long working day, who wouldn't rather go home and flop on the sofa; on a freezing December morning, who wouldn't prefer to stay in bed? In that way, every run is a tiny victory.

I'm no good at collective exercise either. Partly it's self-consciousness, partly it's impatience: standing around waiting for a class to start, waiting for the treadmill to become free, sizing up other gym-goers, all the posturing and posing in front of mirrors. Also, for me there's something depressing about exercising indoors, like a hamster on a wheel. I don't live anywhere particularly scenic, but there are streets, parks, canals. Fresh air. I have friends who actually get in the car and drive to the gym, which seems crazy to me.

My mother – superslim and fit – does not own a tracksuit, shorts or leggings. Whether it's a generational thing, or just her temperament, I don't know, but I can't even picture her in a gym. I was reminded of my elegant, anti-gym mother recently when I read Joanna Lumley's characteristically outspoken views in the *Daily Mail*:

'I don't go to gyms, but I do rush about. I don't like exercising. I find it offensive. People pay money to go and walk on the spot. It disgusts me actually. Go and pick up litter instead. Go and paint an old woman's house. I find gyms oppressive and frightening.' Instead of the treadmill, Lumley says she walks everywhere – and: 'I don't gorge myself. On a typical day I eat lettuce, followed by some lettuce, with lettuce.'

Fortunately for the fitness industry, views like Lumley's aren't fashionable; in fact gyms are very big business. My friend S is a member of four gyms: his gym at home in Glasgow, the gym in his London apartment building, the gym at the University where he works, and the gym in the City where he plays squash. We worked out that it's costing him over £400 a month to feel guilty about not exercising. There are thousands of others like him, who pay for but never use their gym subscription. As S says, 'It makes me feel fitter to be a member, even if I haven't gone for months.'

And the landscape of gyms is rapidly evolving. I recently visited a Fitness First near me, opposite St Paul's in the City of London. No longer a few mouldy treadmills and a corner for the weight-lifters – this gym was like some Orwellian vision of the twenty-first century. Despite the fact that I only wanted to see the swimming pool, the rippling young Aussie insisted on showing me over the entire premises. In a gym the size of an aircraft hangar there were rows of flashing machines and digital monitors, runners and cross-skiers wired up to their heart-rate monitors and calorie-calculators, cyborg-shaped men sculpting their muscles on complicated weight-lifting devices, women on Power Plates having their body-fat vibrated away.

Despite the recession, it seems that a lot of people are still willing to pay over the odds for someone else to help them get thin: I saw several personal trainers sculpting their clients into 'superbodies'. And in the studios, the list of classes was endless: Boxercise, Zumba, Ceroc, BodyPump and FabAbs. Remember when classes meant aerobics?

Gone are those days of gentle stretching, Legs, Bums and Tums with a friendly Jane Fonda video, or *Fame* dance workouts. These days it's all about torching your belly fat, chiselling your muscles, sweating your way to a rock-hard six-pack. Classes are conducted to pumping music, dancing, boxing or spinning till you drop. As my female friend C says, 'When I'm in the gym I'm not even checking out the men. I just want to be more hardcore than the women next to me – run faster for longer, press more weights. I watch what the personal trainers do and I try to do it harder.' It's as though we decided to channel all the dissatisfaction or dislike we feel for our bodies into our workouts.

If I were rich I'd hire a personal trainer three times a week, to take me to the park and make me do lunges and circuits and press-ups on benches. You know, boot-camp stuff. In London, fashionable twenty-somethings sign up to British Military Fitness, army-style training sessions of burpees and hot potato squats led by ex-military types.

Boot-camps are popular with female celebrities, especially those with a fitness DVD to promote. Dressed in crop-top, hot pants and full make-up, and accompanied by a personal trainer, they will go through the motions of a hardcore session in their local park. The relevant media will be informed in advance, and the celebrity will be snapped in a variety of poses. Never mind the hair extensions or the false nails, this is an excellent way to launch their new DVD or beauty line.

I've reviewed a few female fitness camps for magazines: twenty-mile hikes before dawn and clear-broth-for-every-meal kind of places. On one 'weight-loss' retreat in Austria, women were actually sneaking out at night to buy chocolate from the local town. Even for me the memories of that week are pretty miserable. No wonder there was so much crying.

Nevertheless these 'wellness breaks' continue to grow in popularity (despite the fact that any progress made in a week is likely to be undone quite quickly). The short-term nature doesn't seem to matter. Trimmer You, a residential weight-loss camp in the UK, caters specifically to women 'looking to shed post-baby weight, get in shape for an upcoming wedding, tone up for a beach holiday...' Their fitness packages range from 'bikini' to 'bridal'. The testimonials on their website are gushing and grateful: 'My greatest accomplishment? Just knowing that I had pushed through the pain threshold and kept going. I was the biggest girl at my camp but I managed to lose 17 pounds.' GI Jane Bootcamp is another one promising, 'You will lose weight and inches; we guarantee you will drop a dress size in a week.' In America you can take part in prison boot-camps to really whip yourself into shape.

Although I avoid collective exercising I make an exception for kick-boxing. It's intensely hard work, and I hate it and I love it: perhaps an impulse familiar to many of us, that of pushing through the pain barrier, drawing on our deepest reserves, and feeling completely spent by the end. The poster on the wall opposite where we hit the deck, and feint, and box, and skip and jump reads: *What You Gonna Do: Toughen Up or Wimp Out?* And when I come out of my 90-minute kick-boxing session, my face is a deep magenta, and I feel more 'worked-out' than I do after any other exercise I've ever tried. I feel Chizzled Hard as my instructor would say. Why would anyone bother with yoga when they could be perfecting their roundhouse kick?

*

Ah yoga. Something I have been recommended by so many people. Something I have spent decades telling myself I will master. Why oh why do yoga and I just not get on? In the interests of research – out of curiosity, and in the hope that it might change my mind,

I decided to review a new Hot Yoga studio in Islington for my weekly *Times* column.

This week's new experience: my first Hot Yoga class. I'm always hearing about the miracles of yoga, how it brings inner peace and stillness, and I've often wondered if mindfulness could be the crucial element in my recovery.

Well. The studio was heated to about 100 degrees. Around twenty of us gathered, all in tight, strappy yoga gear – I was in my best Sweaty Betty – clutching bottles of water, colourful mats and towels. A Japanese woman at the front of the class massaged Tiger Balm slowly into her temples while omm-ing under her breath, then embarked on a series of yogi-contortions. A few blokes shuffled in, bare-chested in just running shorts, posing in front of the full-length mirror.

The class itself was fine: uncomfortably hot, but I was disappointed at how physically un-taxing it was. I do calisthenics at home every evening, and most of the Hot Yoga moves were quite similar to this – basic suppleness, stretching and strengthening exercises. There wasn't any Sanskrit chanting or breathing: I'd been hoping it would expand my mind as well as my body and leave me spiritually uplifted.

No spiritual uplift for me, sadly. Perhaps I need to persevere, or perhaps we're all looking for something different from our workouts. I need heart-pumping, red-faced, breath-busting cardiovascular exercise. Have you seen the cyclists at the Tour de France, scaling those Alpine peaks? To me, that's the perfect workout; physical exertion so intense that it stills the anxious thoughts. Hot Yoga didn't help my whirring brain at all.

I know what yoga-devotees will say – oh, you should have tried Ashtanga or Kundalini or Iyengar. Sure enough, my friend

L texts me: 'Maybe Hot Yoga isn't for you. You should try something more dynamic – come to Vinyasa with me next week?' L is a personal trainer and all-round fitness fanatic: whenever we meet for coffee she turns up in a tracksuit, her rucksack stuffed with boxing gloves, on her way to train a client. Her professional language includes phrases like 'kill it'.

The Hot Yoga changing room was interesting, from the perspective of female research and seeing what real bodies look like (very unlike magazines). Women casually stripping off, sharing showers, towelling their hair dry while naked. Some women have basic undies and get dressed without much fuss, others use multiple beauty products and spend ages styling their hair and re-applying cosmetics.

I feel a bit uncomfortable showering with all those naked women. Is it just that the changing rooms are highly mirrored so all I can see, at every angle, is breasts and bottoms? Everyone's pretending to be oh-so-natural, while covertly comparing bodies. Oddly, I don't mind communal changing rooms – I have no problem trying on clothes around other women. I'm happy to go topless on the beach, and I've never felt self-conscious about undressing in front of a boyfriend.

Chatting to my friend H about this, I'm reminded how different the Europeans are about nudity: 'When I lived in Germany and went to the local spa, all the women wandered around starkers with no shame,' she said. 'I think it's quite a British/American thing to be so uptight about how we look naked in public.' I had this experience on a ski trip in Austria too: in the steam room at our hotel, my boyfriend and I were glared at for keeping our towels neatly wrapped around our waists.

For now, I'll stick to running and the occasional session of kick-boxing. Yoga seems to promise more than it delivers – for me. The best thing about the whole experience was leaving the hot-box of a studio and cycling home in a gentle breeze. And I have to admit, I slept like a baby that night.

*

Aside from the changing room we don't often see other women's real bodies. Of course naked women are everywhere in the media – models or porn stars, airbrushed and digitally perfected so they appear to have no skin blemishes or cellulite, no sagging breasts or large nipples or bushy pubic hair. You may have seen the 2012 film *Take This Waltz*. Starring Michelle Williams, it was a fairly standard bittersweet romantic comedy, but it hit the headlines for the now-infamous 'shower scene'. There was no horror or porn involved in this shower, but it was discussed in every review I read of the film.

Six women, ranging in age from around thirty to seventy, different shapes and ethnicity, standing in the showers at a municipal swimming pool. But here's the thing: their bodies are not perfect. Some are overweight, most are saggy, all have pubic hair. They chat to each other as naturally as if they were clothed. They shave their legs, they wash their hair, their feet. They are not digitally altered, and they are not movie-star-beautiful. *The New Yorker* referred to their 'pudgy corpulence'.

It's a very naturalistic scene, and yet I (and many critics) found it strangely unnatural. We are used to the casual, ever-present appearance of flawless female flesh to promote products, to sell sex, or fashion, or cars, or diets; it's almost as though 'real' bodies are taboo. Anticipating this, the director Sarah Polley explained: 'I find it really offensive that women's bodies are either objectified or used for comic value.' *The New York Times* said the nudity reminds us that 'young flesh will age; old flesh was once young; time wins in the end'.

Yes, it's something like that. It is unusual, and quite moving, to look at normal women's bodies, but it can also be challenging. It's quite a twisted situation we've got ourselves in. We're used to nudity from toned and tanned body doubles, or perfect Hollywood sex scenes. That doesn't bother us. But being confronted with normal (imperfect) female bodies just washing between their legs or shaving their armpits makes us feel awkward: how did we get so disconnected from reality? As Eva Wiseman wrote in *The Observer*, 'anything other than perfection rings bells'. Our visual culture is full of female nudity, but none of it is genuine. The imperfection of those saggy bellies and breasts seemed to stand for something other than the usual magazine or movie version of titillation.

The male friend I was watching the film with admitted he found it a shock to see normal women naked on-screen. 'Really unusual. None of them were perfect in a Hollywood sense… but I actually preferred it. They were actually much more sexy.' I liked this, and I understood what he meant. An actual woman's body is more exciting – more challenging, and more erotic – than the airbrushed, pornified version could ever be.

*

As it happens, the women in *Take This Waltz* had been participating in gently comic session of aqua-aerobics. And they were enjoying themselves. That in itself is unusual, because for most women, exercise is not about enjoyment. Although we may enjoy exercise, the main reason for exercising is simple: to lose weight, or to maintain an 'acceptable' body-shape. Not to play, as in the original sense of 'sport', nor even to be fitter or healthier or faster. The over-riding point of exercising is to get thinner.

Even the most intrepid women are not immune from the female mind-set which views physical exercise through the prism of weight-loss. In 2012 I heard an edition of Radio 4's *Midweek* in which the explorer Felicity Aston discussed her solo trek across the Antarctic. Libby Purves concluded the interview: 'Finally, most important question, how much weight did you lose?!' Aston replied: '... it was the best diet in the world. I was eating chocolate and jelly beans all day long, and by the end of the expedition I'd lost about a stone.' Obviously it was a light-hearted question, but it has curiously female connotations. Would it have been asked of Captain Scott, Sir Ranulph Fiennes or Bear Grylls?

It's hard to find a single female fitness magazine that doesn't focus on weight and shape: they assess all forms of exercise in terms of calories burned, inches lost and body-fat reduced. As always, with women, it's about shrinkage. Even *Health and Fitness* magazine, which might be expected to emphasise the benefits of exercise, uses the same old terms of body-hatred: *Blitz that Belly! Get a Flat Tum for Life! Fight Fat and Win! Ditch the Love Handles!* A recent *Zest* headline promises: *Slim and Sexy in Six Weeks!*

A 2012 issue of *Top Sante* reported on 'the most extreme workout ever'. How could I resist reading more? Fresh from New York City, the new extreme fitness craze is called SoulCycle. Note that we must be 'extreme' and 'hardcore' these days. Normal is no good. And, from the website, it's clear that SoulCycle is not for your average civilian: the homepage proclaims Athlete-Legend-Warrior-Renegade-Rockstar.

Here's how it works: 'Each SoulCycle ride delivers an intense FULL-BODY workout with a fun and energizing atmosphere. SoulBands is our REVOLUTIONARY class that challenges the entire body by using resistance bands that hang above each bike. Not only do riders burn calories and get their hearts pumping, they also work their core and use hand weights to tone their upper bodies. The 60-minute workout includes several anaerobic intervals and trains the WHOLE body, toning the abs, obliques, shoulders, triceps, biceps and back – all while maintaining fat-burning cardio levels.'

And it's a spiritual workout too, with candles and everything! 'SoulCycle incorporates a mental component of inspirational coaching. By keeping the lights low and riding by candlelight, SoulCycle creates a cardio sanctuary where riders can come to clear their heads.'

The website shows exercise bikes with a system of pulleys and ropes above – not dissimilar to a medieval torture rack. Exhausted riders are pictured stretching the upper half of their body while frantically pedalling with the lower half. The banner headline confidently invites you to… *Take Your Journey. Change Your Body. Find Your Soul.*

I'm not sure about finding your soul – but if you can avoid the motivational clap-trap, being active is definitely worthwhile. Walking around the block on a rainy Sunday evening will cheer you up. Throwing a ball for a dog in the park will put a smile on your face. However low you feel, doing something is better than doing nothing. Exercise makes you feel more positive, even if you don't lose weight. As Juvenal said, '*Mens sana in corpore sano*', a sound mind in a healthy body. Countless studies have shown that exercise is a powerful antidepressant releasing endorphins and boosting mood. And even if you're mentally balanced, perfectly sane, and never lurch from dejection to despair? Well, you might just find it fun.

During the London 2012 Olympics *The Sun* offered the following helpful guide to its female readers:

- Gymnastics – the waist whittler – burns 315 calories an hour
- Diving – the belly buster – burns 197 calories an hour

- Archery – the bingo-wings banisher – burns 238 calories an hour
- Athletics – the all-rounder – burns 590 calories an hour
- Beach volleyball – the bum booster – burns 472 calories an hour

In a post-Olympics article in *The Guardian*, journalist Homa Khaleeli asked why women can't be allowed to enjoy sport for how it makes us feel, rather than how it makes us look. She quoted several women who, on joining a gym, were asked by the staff which areas of their bodies they wanted to work on and where they wanted to lose the inches; even if they simply wanted to get stronger and healthier, train for a triathlon or join classes with friends. Khaleeli concluded: 'The message to women is clear; what matters is not your health or enjoyment, but your weighing scales.'

Khaleeli interviewed Sue Tibballs from the campaign group Women's Sport and Fitness Foundation, who agrees: 'It feels like all the negative energy we put into trying to control our bodies with diets, corsetry and surgery is driven by not liking ourselves – we are really undoing ourselves at the moment by battling our bodies.' Yes, we're battling; waging this one-person war against unsightly lumps, bumps and love handles. Is it any wonder that we feel disgust towards ourselves, when we are harangued from all sides with gym-guilt, reminded of the virtues of trimming down, toning up, getting rid of our excess flesh? My friend C told me:

> *At the start of every month I promise myself: three nights a week I'll go the gym. Come on, just three nights, just for 30 minutes. And then I make excuses, and Tuesday becomes Friday and I've only gone to the gym once or not at all, and when I don't go, I sit on the sofa eating and feeling shit about myself. And guilty every time a beautiful, slim, fit woman appears on TV. And I don't understand how not-going can make me hate myself so much.*

Whether we exercise or not, it shouldn't make us feel guilty. Children run and jump because they can; because it feels good. Maybe C is slightly stuck in a negative pattern, trying to force herself to the gym – but I know how she feels. As women, we're so weighed down with the sense of should and could: I *should* be working out, I *could* be slim if only I wasn't so lazy/greedy – that we end up doing nothing. It's the most pointless form of self-sabotage, and one we're all familiar with.

Are we really going to spend our whole lives like this, feeling the wrong shape and the wrong weight in the wrong skin? Watching the Paralympics recently made me feel quite ashamed: we should never, whether we have all our limbs intact, or some of them missing, with disabilities, abnormalities or simple imperfections, hate our own bodies. We should not allow the gym to become a grim regime of pain and punishment. Maybe we could try, idealistic as it sounds, to find something we love; to regain the joy in simple movement; to be happy minds in healthy bodies.

*

'Go hard or go home.'

Sometimes, it seems, you literally have to go home. This is what happened to me around a decade ago. I was in my third year at Oxford, facing the double challenge of taking my Finals in English Literature while trying to stay out of hospital/eating disorder clinic/loony bin. I was also at my lowest weight with anorexia – around five and a half stone.

In my memory it was winter, January or February, although it seemed to be always winter during the Oxford years. The cold wasn't just outside, and it couldn't be solved with a hat and scarf: it penetrated the marrow of my bones, freezing me from inside. I was taking two or three scalding-hot baths a day to try to generate some body heat; I was eating almost nothing. My bones were covered in livid bruises from the slightest knock; my tailbone ground against the bathtub.

I was up earlier than usual that Sunday morning and crossed the road to the Iffley Road gym (where Roger Bannister ran the first ever four-minute mile). The gym was deserted, and I plugged in my headphones, and did my usual hour on the treadmill, then a couple of kilometres on the rowing machine. On the way out, the gym manager stopped me at the front desk and asked to have a word. They were sorry, he explained, but they had decided to terminate my membership. It was on health grounds, he explained; they would of course refund my remaining months; they felt perhaps I was overdoing it, perhaps I should give my body a rest. I have never been so humiliated in my life.

I still sting from that humiliation, but it was a turning point. Whatever the reasons – self-preservation, vanity, desperation, pride – I gradually managed to gain some weight. It took many years – more than ten – to get to where I am now, which is a normal weight and a healthy Body Mass Index.

That was long ago – I'm allowed in gyms these days. But I think the experience scarred me: I still avoid group activities and I still avoid gyms. And it's probably why I've always chosen solitary forms of exercise: cycling, running, swimming. You're moving too fast, or underwater, for anyone to approach you… These days, running in just a vest top and shorts, I can enjoy the fact that my body looks fit and strong. I remember how people used to look at me with that expression: *You're so thin, why are you running?* There are many good reasons to overcome anorexia, but being free of those glances of pity is one of the best.

*

Olympic athletes are great role models... We live in an age which is constantly about looks and now we're watching bodies that are running fast and jumping high. Suddenly, worrying about 'Am I thin?' seems as silly as it is.

(Dr Linda Papadopoulos, psychologist, in *The Guardian*.)

The slogan for the London 2012 Olympic Games was 'inspire a generation'. And cheesy as it sounds, it did. All of us, even the most ardent sport-sceptics, were caught up in the euphoria. My parents were in France for the entire summer; like many people they were happy to escape the Olympics. And yet, when they rang to sympathise with me for being 'stuck in London', I found myself trying to convey the magical atmosphere. I wasn't stuck, the traffic wasn't gridlocked, and the transport system didn't collapse, as had been predicted. Cycling to work, the roads were deliciously free of cars: it felt liberating, like the cyclists had taken over the capital. The streets weren't thronged with tourists, in fact the centre of London was deserted because everyone had gone east, to Stratford. There were no terrorist bombs or threatened attacks; none of the terrible security delays came to pass.

Like most of the UK I didn't get tickets, and yet I felt part of the Games. I don't own a television, but I found myself compulsively watching the important events (i.e. anything involving Jessica Ennis) on the BBC iPlayer. Each day, more Olympic Gold medals were swept into our basket; each day a new champion was born. In every newspaper, journalists asked: what will we do when it's over?

It's hard to pinpoint what was so special: the sun shone, it was our golden summer, we were united, basking in the media spotlight, welcoming the outside world, waving our flags. And London looked so beautiful: we were proud of ourselves. And it wasn't just London – all over the UK, for two spellbinding weeks during the Olympics, and then another two weeks during the Paralympics, we were all part of Team GB.

Social media played an important part in the fun too. On Twitter, even the loneliest of us felt less alone. I was having a tumultuous summer, feeling emotionally fragile, but I was buoyed up by the collective joy of my fellow tweeters (many of them total strangers). I watched the Olympic opening and closing ceremonies in my bathrobe, tweeting away, and it felt like there was an entire party going on in my flat.

As well as these unexpected moments of 'connection', and the outpouring of national pride, there was much excitement about the female athletes. From Olympic boxer Nicola Adams to Paralympic swimmer Ellie Simmonds, women were in the media spotlight for their strength and determination, not for their latest breast surgery or the footballer they were dating. They had worked for their success, they were famous as a result of hard graft and athletic prowess, not just for being famous. They were winners, not airheads.

A 2012 study by the Women's Sport and Fitness Foundation found that, although eight-year-old girls did a similar level of activity to boys (60 per cent engaging in physical activity for at least an hour, five days a week) by the time girls reached fourteen that figure had halved. The teenage girls questioned said they didn't like exercising in front of boys, did not feel confident about their sporting skills, and viewed sweating as unfeminine. 'At present only 12 per cent of fourteen-year-old girls do the level of activity recommended by the government and nearly half say they lack sporting role models', reported *The Sunday Times* in July 2012.

So, positive Olympic role models for girls? Female empowerment sorted, sexist struggle over – job done? Well, not exactly. Whilst I agree that it was refreshing to see women using their bodies for sporting excellence rather than as sex objects, and valued for their physical rather than purely aesthetic qualities, there was lots of ogling going on.

Look at the beach volleyball debacle: a more puerile example of schoolboy sniggering among grown men would be hard to find. Sample conversation among my male friends, brothers and colleagues: 'Did you apply for tickets?' 'Yeah, for girls' beach volleyball.' 'Good one mate.' 'Yeah <snigger, snigger>' The volleyball arena was situated on Horseguards Parade, not far from the Houses of Parliament. On Radio 4 I heard several male politicians cracking jokes about supporting Team GB by spending a day at the beach volleyball, or how the Prime Minister could just about glimpse the arena from the back of 10 Downing Street. The volleyball players competed in bikinis, and the men were entranced. Women were highly visible, and minimally clad.

(Really, is there any technical reason why female volleyball players or javelin throwers should compete in sporty bikinis, when their male counterparts wear T-shirts and shorts? In almost every athletic discipline women are exposing far more flesh than men.)

I did not spend the entire summer fuming like this. Along with the rest of the country, I was enthralled by the rowers and the gymnasts, the footballers and the swimmers, both female and male. But I am not convinced that our summer of female champions heralds a new era for women. The Olympic athletes are super-fit – and although this is through their own training, rather than cosmetic surgery or radical diets, still their muscular perfection is unachievable for most women. My friend C said, 'Those Olympic bodies make me feel even worse about myself than skinny models in magazines do.'

And anyway, appearance *does* come into it. While the Olympics and the Paralympics showcased a wide range of female athletes, it's the prettiest of them who have become the real stars. Jessica Ennis and Victoria Pendleton had already bagged lucrative beauty campaigns (with Olay and Pantene) before they won gold at London 2012. The open-water swimmer Kerri-Anne Payne did not win an Olympic medal in 2012 but she is the face of Max Factor and Oral B, among other lucrative sponsors. Plenty of other women who *did* win gold medals in the Olympics and Paralympics weren't signed up by the advertising scouts, presumably because they're not deemed physically perfect enough. In Team GB, as in life, it's the glamour girls who do best.

Throughout the Games the media focused relentlessly on the barely clothed female form – how could it not? The Team GB outfits designed by Stella McCartney were eye-wateringly tiny, often causing female athletes to expose one or both buttocks when they ran or jumped or vaulted. Their bodies were tanned, toned and completely hairless (during the gymnastics there was plenty of tweeting going on about the amount of hot wax these athletes must get through). It is true that those women were not there because of their looks – but their looks were amazing. The obsession with Jessica Ennis's six-pack sparked an explosion in bookings for abdominal cosmetic surgery, according to one Harley Street clinic. I lost count of the number of magazine articles about how to 'Get Jess's Rock-Hard Abs'. Many of the swimmers competed in full eye-make-up ('must be ferociously waterproof' one friend tweeted) and athletes of every discipline had their nails manicured with the Union Jack.

Let's be honest, it wasn't hard to feel positive about women during London 2012. For once, female sport was receiving proper coverage – far more than the annual ration of tiny skirts on long-limbed tennis stars at Wimbledon – but the balance was short-lived. In October 2012, The *Daily Telegraph* reported that the

Olympic Games legacy risked not doing enough to promote women in sport – despite the success of Team GB female athletes at the London 2012 Games.

Normal service has already resumed on television, with blanket coverage of football, rugby, cricket and golf, all male. Outside the Olympics only 5 per cent of media coverage is dedicated to female sport. All-female matches receive just 0.5 per cent of all commercial sponsorship, and only one in five board members of national sports governing bodies are women. The Women's Sport and Fitness Foundation reports that 'The under-promotion and underfunding of women's sport is leading to an "inactivity crisis" among women, with just 20 per cent of females currently doing enough exercise to benefit their health.'

So it's debatable whether London 2012 really marked a sea-change in the battle for gender equality. During the games, a couple of posters on *The Guardian* website discussed this:

> *Don't want to sound cynical but I bet you a tenner the effect of the powerful female will disappear within a week and we'll be back to the usual promotion of attractive women as stick-thin insects with child-like frames.*

Another wrote:

> *So now we have to spend 6 hours a day in the gym to meet the new muscular body shape? What's changed here then?*

Exactly – the focus is still on women's bodies. Despite the fact that female athletes (presumably) never set out to be supermodels, they're still judged on their size. If it's not the media itself, there is the endless barrage of body-bashing from the public court of the Internet. As the website www.nationalpost.com commented, 'there's nothing like anonymity to bring out the woman-hater in us all'.

The British world and Olympic champion swimmer Rebecca Adlington has frequently spoken of the derogatory online comments and abusive Twitter messages she receives: 'It is awful and I get angry. Most things that I read about myself are not swimming related. They are to do with how I look, which has nothing to do with my performance in the pool.'

The Australian swimmer Liesel Jones was also subjected to body-criticism during the Olympics, with headlines such as 'Is she fat, or is this what fit looks like?' all over the Internet. *The Huffington Post* ran an article entitled 'Fat and Fearless?' A fellow swimmer commented: 'Leisel has never had that tiny straight up and down, very sinewy, lean swimmer's body and she's managed to win countless amounts of Olympic and Commonwealth Games medals.' Fortunately Jones herself wasn't bothered by her lack of washboard abs; she said the criticism was 'the best thing that happened to me: you put me under pressure and I'll show you what I can do'.

It seems all sportswomen are fair game, even our national treasures. Jessica Ennis, physically sublime by most people's standards, was judged to be 'fat' by certain members of the UK Athletics hierarchy, as was the heptathlete Louise Hazel. Female athletes are being evaluated on aesthetic standards that have nothing to do with their sporting ability. They would not be fast or strong or powerful if they were stick-thin; they could not win medals if they were underfed. The Olympic triathlete Hollie Avil quit the sport at the age of twenty-two after suffering from an eating disorder (which she claims was triggered by a remark made by a British Triathlon coach about her weight).

When will we start to encourage and value women, as we do men, for their creative, intellectual and non-physical abilities;

for their brains not their bodies? While the buzz around female Olympians was a welcome change, they hardly represent your 'average' woman. Young, chiselled, minimally clad, gold-medal winners may be inspirational, but they are also impossibly perfect in their own way.

So, new models of femininity? The end of the skinny supermodel, the size-zero actress and the surgically enhanced reality TV star; the dawn of the strong and muscular female form? As powerful and beautiful as they are, ironically these Olympian women may simply have given us another reason to feel inadequate about ourselves. We could just end up replacing one unattainable body ideal with another.

Chapter 6

THE MINISTRY OF FASHION AND BEAUTY

Welcome to the Ministry of Fashion and Beauty (FAB). Now that you're on the road to thin, you'll want to look the part. From clothes, to shoes, to body hair, to cosmetics, the perfect body is nothing without perfect styling.

Fashion is a twenty-first century minefield: what to wear in your twenties, forties, or sixties; how to style yourself for day, or work, or evening, or holidays. Even if you're still struggling – even if you still have a few kilograms to lose – don't worry: there is a way to dress that will conceal all your physical imperfections. Pear or apple-shaped; muffin topped or bingo-winged; the right clothes can hide a multitude of body crimes.

But don't think you can make it up. Don't think that wearing your favourite boot-cut jeans from a few years ago, or a simple Little Black Dress with sparkly earrings, or wedge heels, or a pencil skirt is OK, because it's not. Fashion is constantly evolving and the rules change all the time. And anyway, no one with chunky thighs should ever wear knee-high boots – *what were you thinking?*

Let's be honest: supermodels on the runway look amazing. But can you imagine actually replicating the runway trends: wearing a conical bra outside your shirt, maybe, or a skirt made entirely of feathers, or a cat on top of your head? Walking to the train station or the shops in 6-inch spike heels and latex leggings? Of course fashion shows shouldn't be taken too seriously – they're a spectacle, a theatrical fantasy. Normal women couldn't wear that kind of haute couture, even if they could afford it.

There is a huge disconnect between us and them, which brings us back to the all-powerful Ministry of Thin. Most models are not only young and beautiful, but also extremely slim. A female fashion editor I know, in her fifties, says: 'Sure the clothes are bizarre – but the girls are so skinny they get away with it.' Because that's the truth: fabric hangs well on frames which are straight up-and-down. No bumps, no lumps or unsightly flab. Nothing to get in the way of the designer's artistic vision.

The average woman wears around 20 per cent of her wardrobe around 80 per cent of the time. We stick to neutral colours – black, white, navy – and we play it safe. While many of us enjoy flicking through fashion magazines, and occasionally even splashing out on gorgeous outfits, on the whole we stick to what works. We wear clothes that cover the 'shameful bits', enhance the good bits, and make us look slimmer. 'Does my bum look big in this?' needs no explanation, ever... The fashion and beauty rules, like so many female rules, are driven by the underlying principle that thinner is better.

When it comes to the FAB rules, few women get it right. Most of us get it wrong, wrong, wrong. So what should we wear? What make-up should we buy? Is it OK to just buy clothes we like; is it better to try or not to try at all: are we too fat for them, or too old?

Make no mistake, the FAB rules matter.

*

The FAB rules are hard to follow, and even harder to predict. I remember when trainers with wedge heels appeared a few years ago, they were mocked as tasteless – now they're supercool. And look at the transition from boot-cut jeans to skinny jeans: the first were designed to even out your silhouette, the second cling to every curve. Then there are those inexplicable trends: piling all your hair up in a top-knot – sorry, the 'messy high bun' – or ankle socks worn with high heels. On about 99 per cent of us, these look ridiculous. What are we trying to say, when we shop, or dress, or apply our make-up?

A hundred years ago 'nice' girls didn't paint their faces; now women of all social classes use fake tan and false eyelashes. I loved this recent *Sunday Times* snippet from the novelist Fay Weldon: 'When I was young, nice girls covered up. I buttoned my sleeves at the wrist and my collar up to the neck. Skirts were mid-calf. Stockings were lisle. Court shoes, black or brown. Make-up was minimal. Lipstick was rose for good girls, scarlet for bad.'

The distinction between 'good' and 'bad' girls barely exists these days; in fact, haute couture is often a subversion of 'chav' culture. White stilettos and handbags are making a comeback. It's fine to dress like a prostitute, as long as you do it ironically. High-society models such as Alice Dellal shave the sides of their head and wear ripped fishnet stockings while advertising luxury brands. For decades, animal prints in any form were considered trashy – now a nice, expensive pair of leopard-print ballet pumps or trousers adds a touch of class.

Perhaps it's no surprise that we're uncertain how we should look, when we're bombarded with constant advertising for clothes, shoes and cosmetics. You don't need to live anywhere near the shops these days to be a consumer: the Internet enables you to spend money 24/7. And yet, the more we spend, the less it seems to fill us up: like a low-fat, low-calorie diet which leaves you constantly hungry.

Shopping can be a kind of itch. Sometimes I'll realise I haven't bought anything for a few days, and buying something, even just a few magazines in Tesco, seems to relieve this. For many women shopping no longer needs a specific purpose – to find a birthday gift or replace a pair of shoes – it's a leisure activity, something to fill the days. We sort of browse aimlessly, flick through the rails, wait for something to catch our eye. Sometimes when I'm out shopping with friends, flicking though the rails of jeans – skinny jeans, boyfriend jeans, high-cut jeans, ultra-low-rise – it dawns on me that I can't actually picture what is already in my wardrobe. The whole retail experience induces a kind of brain fog. Just now, for an experiment, I counted up how many jeans I own – all of them, not just the ones I wear. Thirty-one pairs. And I'm not even a fashionista.

I could try to make excuses – I don't wear most of those jeans, some of them are really dated, and the designer pair which I love are ripped under the bum so I had to replace them. And anyway, post-anorexia, it's inevitable that I'll have a lot of different sizes of clothing, ranging from size tens to size zeros. But that's rubbish and I know it. Thirty-one pairs of not wildly dissimilar jeans is Far Too Many.

In Chapter 1 I mentioned the food rationing during the Second World War. On the same website I was fascinated (and appalled, given my jeans census) by the equally frugal clothing allowance. Here's the deal: from June 1941 every individual was allocated 66 clothing coupons a year – which equated to roughly one complete outfit. (Later in the War, the allocation was cut to only 48 coupons.) The following list illustrates the number of coupons needed to buy certain garments:

- Woman's nightdress = 6 coupons
- Man's overcoat = 16 coupons
- Dress = 11 coupons
- Underpants = 4 coupons
- Handkerchief = ½ coupon
- Pyjamas = 8 coupons

This era is where the phrase 'make do and mend' comes from. With such tight restrictions, people repaired and recycled worn-out clothes – for example they unravelled the wool of old jumpers to knit it into socks and scarves for the British troops. In 1942 a utility scheme was introduced to restrict the amount of material used in garments. Women's clothing had to have:

- no elastic waistbands
- no fancy belts, and
- shoes with a maximum heel height of 5 cm

Heels of only 5 cm? Imagine that; how would we cope today? Because if there's one item that really defines modern fashion it's the bizarre footwear. I hesitate to call them shoes because they impede the basic activity of walking. They're more like instruments of torture, insane contraptions designed by misogynists or the devil. They give women cloven hooves.

Apparently British women wear the highest heels in Europe. In order of height, Newcastle's heels come top, with London and the West Midlands in second and third place. This survey was carried out by Compeed, makers of padded foot inserts, and the results are hardly a surprise. Of course Newcastle women wear the highest heels – they also wear mini-skirts and bikini tops to nightclubs in midwinter – Geordie girls are made of tough stuff.

But how high is too high? In the UK we seem to have a talent for getting it wrong. Consider the women of Paris, Barcelona or Milan. They do style, class and understated chic. We do binge-drinking and tottering around in stripper shoes.

It's not that I'm ideologically opposed to women wearing heels. I love an elegant pair of shoes as much anyone, and own stilettos, kitten heels, knee-high boots. But this new breed of extreme platform heel is another matter altogether. To me, they represent everything that we've fought against over the last century and more, liberation, emancipation, the vote. We ditched restrictive corsets and stays, we abandoned fussy petticoats and gloves, then we burned our bras. And now? Women are cramming their feet into blocks of wood in which they can hardly walk, let alone run for the bus or jump for joy. Why don't they just go the whole hog and bind their feet?

This is no exaggeration. Podiatrists say that the continual wearing of high heels with narrow toe space can actually lead to foot deformities, just like Chinese women experienced from foot binding. Prolonged use of extreme heels can cause bunions and curvature of the spine.

So where do these heels come from? Mostly from male fashion designers who are concerned with form not function, a sort of high-heel-one-upmanship: Christian Louboutin and his signature red soles; Manolo Blahnik, Jimmy Choo, Patrick Cox, Salvatore Ferragamo; ever wilder creations and to hell with wearability. I find it a little sinister, men designing excruciating shoes for women. Apparently some actresses at the Oscars have pain-relieving injections in the soles of their feet so they can make it down the red carpet: that's how bad some of these shoes are. When extreme footwear first began to cross from the catwalk onto the high street, the journalist Sarah Sands wrote in *The Independent*: 'They are inhumanly uncomfortable – and yet self-imposed. There is an ecstatic relief at stepping out of them at the end of the day. One gazes down at swollen, red, slashed, blistered feet...'

That's the best moment: taking them off. On the rare occasions I wear painfully high shoes I promise myself, never again. For example, this year's New Year's Eve party, at a friend's apartment overlooking Battersea Power Station. I wore a little black dress, sheer black tights and vertiginous black leather ankle boots, spike heeled, four or five inches. My boyfriend couldn't take his eyes off my legs – desired effect – and yes I felt sexy. The heels were fine at first, getting dolled up at home, even walking to the train station. But after five hours at the party, just standing around with drinks, as you do (on spikes), then walking down to the Embankment to watch the midnight fireworks, then wandering around Chelsea looking for a taxi, I was gritting my teeth with pain. By the time we arrived home every step was agony. I hobbled up the stairs, collapsed in the hallway, almost weeping as I unzipped the boots and cradled my poor feet. The soles were inflamed and blistered, my heels on fire, the elegant black tights in shreds.

I remember almost nothing of the New Year party except the searing pain of those spike heels. I don't want to be that woman again, too crippled by silly footwear to stroll home along the river when there are no cabs. I make myself and everyone around me miserable when my shoes are causing such intense pain. Normally, I prioritise function over form, zipping around town in trainers, ballet pumps or motorbike boots. I feel obscurely guilty when I pass other women 'making the effort' in skyscraper-heels, but I don't understand how they can do it, walking around day after day in virtual stilts. The truth is, I simply can't operate effectively in the world like that.

Of course I understand that looking good isn't comfy. A lack of practicality is sexy. As the French saying goes: *il faut souffrir pour être belle* – a woman must suffer to be beautiful. I get the idea behind the high heel; it elongates the woman's leg, forces her to stand in a certain way, to wiggle provocatively as she walks, buttocks thrust out, chest forward. I know that men love heels in the bedroom. Remember the Yves St Laurent Opium advertisement in 2000, showing Sophie Dahl, naked but for her jewels and heels, legs splayed. Interestingly, this was the eighth most-complained-about advert in the last 50 years, according to the Advertising Standards Agency. People said it was too suggestive; Sophie Dahl said: 'I think the photograph is beautiful... it was seen as being anti-women, when in fact I think it is very empowering to women.'

That e-word – empowering – so often heard in the Ministry of Fashion and Beauty is usually suspect. Extreme platforms give a woman extra height, but authority, power? What could be more ridiculous than women in pain or unable to walk or run, those unsteady figures of fun clinging to each other outside nightclubs. I don't know why I feel so strongly about these heels – perhaps because strolling around is one of the most basic things we do as human beings. I asked a couple of my friends what they think:

> I have only one pair of injuriously high heels which I wear maybe a handful of times a year. I would be lying if I said they didn't make me pleased with the appearance of my legs though.

> I do feel quite glamorous in heels but I feel angry as a feminist that it's thought of as sexy or necessary for women to wear them.

> I hate the idolisation of shoes, the way that women go all 'Ooh I'd do anything for a Jimmy Choo.' They are just shoes! They are supposed to be useful. You should always be able to run in your shoes if you have to.

I have strong negative feelings towards high heels and am consciously trying to wear them less. I am extremely uncomfortable with the position they force your body into, it's sexualisation and another way to limit women's movement...

If we're wearing these ridiculous shoes for men, we might as well not bother. If you ask them, the majority of men would prefer a partner who can walk pain-free, and move naturally, than someone who is wincing with every step. My best male friend put it neatly: 'The right woman in the right shoes standing in a bar looks fabulous, but the image is destroyed when she goes to move, grabs onto her friend and nearly topples over even before she's had a drink! Of course high heels look hot – but a happy girl in trainers looks even better.'

This goes to the heart of the heels debate: how can we live with gusto if our shoes are holding us back? I'm not against high heels on the grounds of sexy, simply on the grounds of mobility.

*

Maybe we shouldn't despair quite yet. The new high heels are extreme, but fashions come and go, right? Perhaps, like ra-ra skirts or fringed jackets, we will look back on 6-inch stripper shoes and smile.

What I don't understand is why the Fashion and Beauty rules take everything that used to be beautiful and exaggerate it until it's ugly: huge silicone boobs, gaudy talons, blindingly laser-white teeth. Tiny differences – even flaws – used to be what made a person individual and irresistible; think of Audrey Hepburn's elfin crop, Twiggy's fragility and her gappy front teeth, Marilyn's audacious curves. In the Ministry of FAB, the new beauty is homogeneous and curiously one-dimensional. Where adverts for bronzers and self-tan used to promise the subtle, sun-kissed look, now they proudly use names such as Fake Bake. There is no pretence of an actual sun-tan, and the result is often an all-over shade of orange or mahogany.

Make-up is more complicated than it used to be: primer, highlighter, fake tan, illuminator, hair extensions, nail art and the rest. I remember the beauty advice in my favourite teenage magazines: *Set your alarm half an hour early so you can sneak out of bed, brush your teeth, comb your hair and apply tinted moisturiser and clear mascara. That way you'll wake up next to your boyfriend looking fresh and glowing!* It's easy to laugh, remembering our furtive early-morning bathroom scurries, all that effort for the 'natural' look. 'Who me? Oh, I just naturally wake up with my breath all minty-fresh.'

There is something ageing about the heavily made-up look, as this anonymous Internet rant points out: 'In my day, putting on so much slap, having a perma-tan, and a massive cleavage was generally reserved for "the older lady" in the same way as women like Dolly Parton, Joan Collins, Barbara Windsor, pile on foundation and primp and preen. I still associate that high level of stage make-up with their generation even though it's the young women doing it now.'

And all that glue: glued-on hair extensions, glued-on eyelashes, glued-on fake nails. I once worked in an advertising agency in New York and one of the women had serious talons, inches beyond her finger ends. They were so long that she click-clacked incessantly on the keyboard and scrabbled to retrieve coins from her purse. Sometimes those extreme talons remind me of corpses, where the nails continue to grow after death.

As with high heels, I have nothing against pretty nails *per se* – I love the occasional manicure and pedicure. But once again, it's the extreme nails, like extreme platforms, which wind me up. The way they impede women going about their daily lives.

Trying to keep up with the new beauty rules is a time-consuming (and expensive) business. Clearly I'm a bad example – I regularly leave the house without mascara, for example – and I have no excuse for this, except my own laziness. I have female friends who make much more of an effort than me: they have their hair trimmed and coloured every six weeks, and they wear a full face of make-up every day, not just for parties. They get waxed regularly – whether they're single, dating or married – and would never dream of going on holiday without a full Brazilian.

*

Oh dear. Brazilians. Just as I was starting to calm down about high heels the body-hair debate rears its head. Here is another one of those beauty issues that seems to have run away with itself: women not being allowed to have ANY body hair. I've just had quite a heated argument with a male friend about female body hair. It went something like this.

Me: *Isn't it terrible, these little girls getting their legs waxed from the age of ten? Don't they realise they have a lifetime of worrying about body hair ahead of them – why start so young?*
S: *I don't know. Nothing wrong with nice smooth legs is there?*
Me: *Of course not, but little girls are not women. They shouldn't be anxious about their appearance at that age – they're becoming sexualised before they even reach their teens. And anyway, who says smooth legs are better?*
S: *Well, women seem to like smooth legs, that's why they shave them.*
Me: *Oh really, that's why we shave? And is that why women are waxing their arms these days? And removing every last scrap of*

pubic hair, like a plastic Barbie doll, a prepubescent child? Do you have any idea how boring it is to shave your legs and underarms every single day?

S: *Come off it, men shave their faces every morning. That's a hassle too.*

Me: *What? How can you compare shaving the bottom half of your face – which by the way, you're not even obliged to do, men are perfectly free to grow stubble or beards – with defoliating half your body? This is just sexist bullshit – women grow hair just like men, and we're wasting our lives endlessly removing it only for it to grow back! Where will it all end?!*

OK I was being strident, but when it comes to female bodies, hair is becoming the ultimate taboo. Is there some perverse logic at work here, where as the hair on our heads grows more lustrous, shiny and bouncy, (ideally with fake extensions) our bodies must be ever more hairless? Smooth legs and underarms are nothing new – *Harper's Bazaar* first advertised hair-removal products for women in 1915.

The bikini wax followed the invention of the bikini in the 1950s, and the Brazilian wax – where nearly all the pubic hair is removed – arrived in the 1980s, along with the thong. But even by the 1990s, when my sisters and I were teenagers, the main preoccupation was still leg and underarm hair. We used razors or Nair – a vile-smelling hair-removal cream – and one friend used Jolen cream bleach on her upper lip. Waxing wasn't the big business it is today – you could buy wax strips for use at home, but most of us abandoned them after painful experiment. (Ripping off the wax strip hurts like hell, which is why you need someone else to do it.) I usually get my legs waxed before summer holidays, and I've always plucked my eyebrows to keep them neat – I find it curiously therapeutic.

After a century of some – not all – women shaving their legs and underarms, the body-hair debate seems to be accelerating. As I mentioned in the Introduction, Julia Roberts' 'underarm hair' moment in 1999 caused uproar among the beauty police. At the film premiere of *Notting Hill*, the actress appeared in a long red dress, waving to fans and exposing unshaven armpits. Afterwards Roberts seemed to be amazed by the fuss, saying: 'On a day-to-day basis I don't think about my armpits.'

If only the rest of us could say the same. A recent UK study found that 99 per cent of women removed some hair, most commonly from the underarms, legs, pubic area and eyebrows. The female population of the UK is now estimated to spend £280m a year removing body hair.

Maybe the worldwide censure of Julia Roberts marked a tipping point: a moment at which women's bodies no longer belonged to them. In truth I think it began long before that, with television and mass media, but the armpit debacle certainly illustrated the vicious power of the Internet to pass judgement. Women with cellulite, sweat-patches, wrinkles or zits have always been fodder for the celebrity magazines; now these images can be shared – and condemned – across the world, instantly. It simply wasn't acceptable for an actress to appear on the red carpet with hair under her arms: really, what was she *thinking*?

Checking images (still all over the Internet) for Roberts' 1999 armpit-fail, I'm amused to see that she's recently dared to do it again. On holiday the 'mother of three' is pictured in a lovely printed bikini, revealing her unshaven armpits – cue cheap headlines such as 'Not afraid to razor controversy' and 'Call in the fashion fuzz'. It takes guts to be a hairy celebrity these days.

Another woman who broke the rules was actress Louise Brealey. She appeared nude *with body hair* on the London stage, as she explained to *The Times*:

I grew my underarm hair because I wanted to be naked on my terms, to make the point that you could be beautiful with hairy armpits. The thing is, women feel like we have a choice about shaving, but we don't. It's a choice between looking normal, and making most potential lovers gag. All but one man I told was openly appalled. But a weird thing happened: I started to like it. When you can see my pubic hair as well, it looks kind of great – like it matches. Like a hat and gloves. Like it's meant to be there.

(*The Times*, December 2012)

(I love this image – 'like a hat and gloves'!)

As the interference into women's bodies spreads, the patches of permissible body hair shrink: we're reaching a tipping point where the removal of all body hair is *de rigeur*. Merran Toerien, a sociologist from the University of York, explains the tangled link between gender and hair on the BBC News website: 'Historically, medically and in the media, hair is nearly always associated with men. Shaving female body hair is seen as a way to differentiate between the sexes. Society dictates that female body hair should be tamed and looked after, women are not allowed to let their bodies just be...'

And that's at the root of it. We sense, instinctively, that women with body hair are perceived as less feminine, more aggressive, less attractive. In the 1970s, not shaving became a feminist statement, an act of defiance.

I can't be the only one who feels that body-hair rules are becoming oppressive. And pornographic. Leg and underarm hair is one thing, but what about the rest of it? It was ever-tinier swimsuits and then thongs which led to the removal of hair along the 'bikini-line' and now pubic hair should not exist. In hardcore online porn, on underwear models, and in increasingly explicit pop videos, the genital area is almost entirely revealed, smooth and hairless. The obvious connotations of pre-pubescence are disturbing enough, that men are aroused by adult women appearing to have the vaginas of little girls.

More than that, it's the incursions into the private space which makes me angry; the purely aesthetic preferences of the porn industry (to make sexual penetration more visible and therefore graphic) and the marketing campaigns of the beauty industry: buy more hair-removal products, waste more time worrying about your appearance, try to look like a porn star. Teenage girls are trying to remove all pubic hair; teenage boys grow up expecting women to be hairless. This zero tolerance to body hair bullshit has trickled into the mainstream, affecting how men view women, naked, and how we feel about ourselves.

I recently took part in a roundtable debate on body image at Channel 4, with female journalists, MPs and broadcasters. One woman related a conversation she'd had with her twenty-five-year-old brother about sex. She mentioned the body-hair issue, and he looked 'confused'. It emerged that he had never had a sexual partner with body hair. Every one of the nine women he'd slept with, in their late teens and twenties, had removed all their pubic hair. Not a single body hair on a single one of his girlfriends. Completely hairless.

It doesn't even make sense. Just because porn stars, and models, and Brazilian beach-bunnies wax everything off, why would we want, or feel obliged, to look like them? Like so many other dictats coming out of the Ministry of Fashion and Beauty, it's pushing women way beyond what is natural.

As I write, 'Armpits for August' is taking place – a group of women bravely abandoning their razors to raise money for charity. A journalist on the *Huffington Post* website is blogging about not shaving for six weeks ('It's The Pits', apparently). I'm not sure what to make of these armpits stunts. It may be the only way we start to address the stigma surrounding female body hair – but it's also slightly depressing. As if women leaving hair under their arms is a political act. Don't we have more important issues to think about, and more powerful ways to communicate the feminist struggle?

On this, and many of the FAB rules, I'm conflicted (and probably hypocritical). As I said in the Introduction, you may prefer to look the way women are supposed to look, hairless and smooth, your skin tanned, your eyebrows neatly groomed. And I do too. But is it really our preference: is it OK to say no?

*

So, extreme platforms, all-over body waxing and miracle lotions and potions – the Ministry of Fashion and Beauty keeps itself busy inventing ever stricter rules for us to follow. And it looks askance at any infringement of these rules. On a recent slow Friday afternoon, browsing the Internet, I discovered this list of beauty blunders...

1. Heavily pencilled eyebrows
2. Foundation marks around the chin
3. Trout pouts
4. Over-plucking of eyebrows
5. Dark lip-liner with pale lipstick
6. Palms of hands going orange from applying fake tan
7. Monobrow
8. Greasy hair
9. Hairy legs
10. Lipstick on teeth
11. Too much make-up
12. Yellow teeth

13. Too much blusher
14. Yellow hard skin on feet
15. Gems stuck onto your tooth
16. Lip-liner outside the edge of the lips
17. Bad hair extensions
18. Clumpy mascara
19. Gelling hair to your face in swirls
20. Pierced finger nails
21. Fake beauty spots
22. Sunburn
23. Roots showing
24. Panda eyes from sunbathing in sunglasses
25. Wearing make-up in bed

Most striking, in my view, is the nastiness of these kinds of lists. You don't need a PhD to know that 'clumpy mascara' isn't ideal, but why must beauty advice take this woman-hating tone? Women's magazines regularly write about fashion crimes – often next to pictures of celebrities with a large tick or a cross, 'What were they thinking?' They do the same with celebrity body parts, or sweat patches, or 'unsightly' rolls of flesh. One publication used to devote an entire page to anonymous photographs of members of the public, snapped out and about, committing fashion no-nos (denim jackets with jeans, or too-short skirts etc.). It's nasty, sneering, vicious. There is a sense that we'd better watch out, that we live in dire risk of committing any one of these 'blunders'. As in so many areas of women's lives, the fashion and beauty police are there to remind us that the way we look in our natural state – without perfectly applied make-up, or on-trend fashion or corrective surgery – is 'wrong'.

Even if you follow the guidance to the letter, don't ever think you can win. The line between beauty and blunder is impossibly thin, and chances are you'll mess up. You have to dye your skin a dark shade of fake tan, but having orange hands is a major fail. You have to wear the latest expensive designer sunglasses, but 'panda eyes from sunbathing' are a disaster. Remember, 'over-plucked eyebrows' are wrong, but the 'monobrow' is also a complete no-no. What's recommended one year is a 'crime' the next – who can keep up? Back in the 1980s pop stars regularly gelled 'kiss curls' to their faces – Lisa Stansfield anyone? Madonna, Gwen Stefani and Lady Gaga have all been praised in the past for their peroxided hair with sexy dark 'roots' but we are told not to even attempt this look.

I emailed these beauty blunders to a couple of female friends to ask if they had even been 'guilty' of any of them. One replied 'I started counting how many of these crimes I'm committing today, but lost count after hairy legs, greasy hair, roots...'

Or, as another friend summed it up: 'Rule one: be beautiful. Rule two: don't be not beautiful.'

Why does any of this matter, you may be wondering. Hirsute or smooth, made-up or bare-faced, surely women have more important things to worry about. For me, that's precisely the point: we do have more important things to worry about than the correct eyebrow shape. If we're serious about our lives and careers, if we care about making a difference to the world in medicine or literature or theatre or politics; if we want to make music or scientific breakthroughs or amazing architecture... if we want to spend time on any of this then we need more time. Less time in the bathroom covered in miracle caffeine-infused cellulite creams, less money in beauty salons with our legs spread having our genitals coated with hot wax and then ripped to shreds.

The average woman looks in the mirror around thirty-eight times a day, and that's not because she's vain. It's because it takes a lot of fiddling to look the way we're supposed to these days: dyeing, plucking and straightening of hair, checking and re-applying of slap. Expectations of men's appearance have increased slightly, but to nothing like the same degree. No one minds a man with grey in his hair or calls it a political act (a male friend of mine went grey in his early twenties and has always had an endless stream of pretty girlfriends). A man is allowed a few days of stubble, facial hair, even wrinkles. A man can still, basically, wash and go.

Not so for women. Whatever your opinion on the beauty business, the rules for women are changing fast. If we don't hold the line, somehow, we're in danger of drifting ever further from reality. I dread a future in which fake tan, eyelashes and hair extensions are expected for all women; where body hair is considered obscene (remember that twenty-five-year-old man who had never seen a naked woman with body hair). To me the debate feels urgent, because the higher the bar is raised, the more unreal and time-consuming the 'look' becomes. It's hard to enjoy life when you're hobbling around on platform heels. It's hard to relax when you're vajazzled up like a porn star.

The fashion and beauty rules can cause misery and even hardship. Women – especially younger, less well-off women – are bankrupting themselves on shoes and handbags costing hundreds of pounds. Add in the 'essential' beauty treatments, iPhones, and the general cost of living, inflation up, wages down, rent and house-prices soaring, and it's not a pretty picture.

The more 'stuff' we have, the less satisfied we seem to be. In retrospect, life before mass consumption (before it really took off in the later twentieth century) seems wonderfully innocent. My godmother (in her seventies) tells me about her wardrobe as a young woman: 'A few blouses and skirts, some frocks for Sundays and parties, and a smart dress for evening... Maybe even some slacks if you were especially daring.' Slacks! A few frocks! Oh the simplicity. She showed me some of her dress-making manuals from the 1950s and they made me feel really sad. There was barely a mention of the female figure, or problematic body parts: the emphasis was on the gorgeous materials, the swish of a silk skirt, the cut of a gown. Clothes were about creativity and colour: indigo blue or deep purple or rose pink. These days fashionistas refer to the 'capsule wardrobe', the classics – you know the standard female uniform, well-cut grey trousers, little black dresses, structured jackets, crisp white shirts, nothing outlandish or mismatched. As the FAB rules have become stricter, the joy and colour has leached out of our wardrobes.

There's no doubt we're in a new era for fashion, with women in their fifties looking as fantastic in skinny jeans as their teenage daughters; but what's mutton and what's lamb? The more we try to follow the FAB rules, the less clear they become. Who knows what we can get away with; who decides what is, in that chilling phrase, *age-appropriate*? Should clothes reflect our personality or our body shape; are we trying to express ourselves, reveal our curves, or conceal our imperfections? Something which should be fun – shopping, dressing up, make-up – has turned into such an intense source of female anxiety and insecurity.

And none of this is necessary. Have we forgotten how beautiful women can naturally be?

Chapter 7

THE MINISTRY OF SEX

Ultimately, it really is all about how you look naked... Modish and stick thin may be best to hang clothes on, but catwalk bodies look deeply unsexy naked. Those bony shoulder blades and door-handle hips are not a turn-on in a bikini. Men are much more forgiving and encouraging about flesh than women are.

(A. A. Gill, *Sunday Times Style* magazine, September 2012)

Slender might be beautiful, but is it attractive to men? A. A. Gill's words are a reminder of how complicated the sex-and-thin debate really is.

Throughout human evolution curvaceousness has been equated with womanliness. Art and culture have long focused on the female body as a source of aesthetic beauty, sexual attractiveness, fecundity, and reproduction. The term 'Rubenesque' describes the sensual, full-figure forms of the Flemish Baroque artist Peter Paul Rubens – exemplified in his 'Venus in Front of the Mirror' of 1614. To modern eyes, Venus looks, well, fat. Even in the twentieth century, aside from a brief fashion for androgyny and boyishness in the 1920s, it was considered desirable for women to have generous breasts, hips and bottoms. It wasn't until the 1960s, with the rise of slender models like Twiggy, that the thinner body shape, and the diet industry, really began to take hold.

We all know what we mean by hourglass figure: think of the *Mad Men* actress Christina Hendricks, or the cartoon character Jessica Rabbit. However, the so-called 'hourglass' figure actually describes quite a specific body composition. The inflection points are the bust, waist and hips. Compared to males, females generally have narrow waists, large buttocks and a wider hip section. Research shows that female waist–hip ratio (WHR) correlates strongly to the perception of attractiveness – women with a 0.7 WHR, that is, a waist circumference that is around 70 per cent of the hip circumference, are consistently rated as more attractive by men across a wide range of cultures. The WHR also correlates closely to female fertility, thereby unknowingly guiding men's evolutionary choices. Consciously or not, this is why men have always interpreted female curves as sexually promising: they are clear biological signs of fertility. Size zero may come and go, but men are hard-wired to seek out flesh.

In this way, thin is the antithesis of sexual invitation. Maintaining a perfect thin body is hard work: it takes mental and physical discipline; a rigid approach to eating; a rigorous approach to exercise. And your desire for sex diminishes when you get very thin. Obviously both extremes are unhelpful – you need a certain level of physical self-esteem and confidence to enjoy sex – and of course anyone of any weight can feel insecure about their body. I can't speak for overweight women, but I do know that being underweight makes you feel about as alluring as an old boot. Why would anyone be horny when they haven't eaten for 24 hours? Sex becomes irrelevant, and uncomfortable, when you're starving.

Interestingly, this applies to both men and women. In the Minnesota Semi-Starvation Experiment of 1944 (discussed in more detail in Chapter 10), a group of healthy young male volunteers were restricted to approximately half of their former calorie intake for a six-month period. One of the notable side-effects of semi-starvation was how the men's libidos ebbed away. Pursuing any kind of romantic or sexual relations with women was too much effort for these young men.

It's not so different for women: when your body weight falls below a critical level, menstruation stops, the uterus shrinks, and your capacity for sexual enjoyment plummets. Extreme dieting messes with your hormones – and sex hormones are among the first to dry up when your body is struggling. I can identify with those Minnesota men: when you're semi-starving, everything else is a colossal effort; your brain is stuck on eating and not-eating, food and hunger.

So the notion that anyone would get skinny to attract the opposite sex is ironic: losing weight clobbers your sex drive and defeats the point of wanting to be thin in the first place.

*

'Being too skinny damages fertility more than obesity.'

This was the conclusion of Dr Richard Sherbahn of the Advanced Fertility Center of Chicago, after carrying out almost 2,500 sessions of IVF over eight years. In our fat-phobic society we hear plenty about the dangers of obesity and the need for women to lose weight before getting pregnant. However, focusing on the health risks of being overweight may mean that the risks of being underweight are ignored. 'It seems the ideal body shape for young women is this overly-skinny physique and women don't understand that there is any concern about this,' Dr Sherbahn said in 2012. He advises that women trying to conceive – naturally or with fertility treatment – should be as close to a healthy Body Mass Index (around 18.5–25) as possible.

In fertility terms, size zero is not good news. As I've mentioned, wanting to conceive was the kick-start for me to overcome anorexia – about the only motivation I could find which might come close to defeating it. Last year, I had managed to gain some weight but after ten years of amenorrhea (absence of menstruation) my periods still hadn't returned. Feeling frustrated at my body's lack of progress, I emailed my psychiatrist about my latest great idea (ha) that I should take fertility drugs. All those skinny celebrities manage to conceive – why shouldn't I pop some Clomiphene too?

His reply reminded me just how crucial body-fat is for the female reproductive system.

It's much better, and healthier, to start your cycle naturally rather than use hormones. It's possible that if you're still doing a lot of exercise, you may have increased your muscle-to-fat ratio, and that can prolong the time, and increase the weight you need, before you get periods. Remember, the body's thinking behind the decision to switch on the ovaries is:

(a) Is there enough energy stored (i.e. fat) to feed a baby through the nine months of pregnancy?

(b) Is there enough fat stored to allow the mother to produce milk after the birth?

My long-suffering shrink was trying to explain that, in a biological sense, women really do need fat. Mother Nature does not care about muscle-tone or skinny jeans or size zeros, not when it comes to making a baby. No amount of fruit or 0% Greek yogurt can substitute for solid reproductive building blocks. My personal war on fat was utterly self-defeating: until I got it through my thick skull that fat was not the enemy, I had no chance of having a baby. (As it turned out, the half stone I'd gained simply wasn't enough to restore menstruation – I needed to gain about a stone. Which I did!)

On top of zapping your libido, low levels of body-fat, typical in female athletes, ballerinas and anorexics, cause a range of physical problems: from amenorrhoea to low oestrogen levels to thin uterus lining (which makes it difficult for an embryo to implant). Biologically the female body can't risk becoming pregnant when it doesn't have enough calories to sustain itself, let alone a new life.

In other words, fat is good for conception. Fat triggers the hormones which trigger ovulation and breast-feeding and maternal feelings. Fat prepares the uterus as a cosy nest for the embryo. Women with generous bosoms and bottoms are seen as more fertile and more nurturing because they are – hence the term 'child-bearing hips'.

*

So, if being thin is not good for health, reproduction, or mating rituals, the question is why we pursue it at all. To me, this is the heart of the matter: are we trying to get thin for the opposite sex? For other women? Or for ourselves?

If our efforts to lose weight are aimed at men, we might as well give up. Overwhelmingly, men do not go for skinny women. Despite the media obsession with impossibly slim supermodels and actresses, there is little evidence that men prefer them. I asked five male friends if they would prefer to sleep with Marilyn Monroe or Twiggy, and they all answered 'Marilyn', instantly. (Estimates vary, but she's reported to have been around a size 14–16.) When I asked the same question between Kate Moss or Kelly Brook, the answer was unanimous – yes, Kelly Brook. Curve-tastic.

Skinny models are a tiny proportion of the population, and there is no evidence that they have happier, more fulfilling relationships or careers than normal-sized women. If anything, they are probably more neurotic, controlling and hungry – with a hefty dose of insomnia on top. The average woman in the UK is a size 16 and they manage to find partners, get married, have families. Clearly, slim doesn't equal content. But we continue to believe that we'll be happier when we lose weight. We've all felt that stab of jealousy as a beautiful slender goddess glides into the pub and men's eyes can't help but follow her... Perhaps male preferences for female body shape are no more logical than our own.

Of course, women in pornography, in films and in magazines are super-slim, but they are also surgically and/or digitally enhanced. These are two-dimensional images of perfection, not the real thing. An ex-boyfriend of mine went out with a 'glamour model' for years, and later described the experience as miserable: 'She was on a permanent diet so we never ate in restaurants; she was always getting her nails done or worrying about her make-up, so we hardly ever went out. And she had massive fake tits which should have been good but actually meant she didn't enjoy sex.'

Not the most gentlemanly language, perhaps, but you can see his point. A woman who is permanently 'perfect' cannot enjoy life with abandon. Driving with the roof down will mess up her hair; splashing in the sea will ruin her make-up; cooking delicious, indulgent food will mess up her diet. From my own experience, I know how detrimental strict dieting is to relationships: so much of love and sex is about food, enjoyment, and letting go. What is more romantic: a candlelit meal or a couple of guilt-ridden Ryvitas?

Men ogle slim women but they don't necessarily want to sleep with them. Women want to wear skinny jeans, but men want something to grab onto. This is what A. A. Gill calls 'the biggest, most fundamental and most important difference in how men and women see women.' There seems to be a disconnect between what women think men want: supermodel-beautiful, and what men really want: Marilyn-voluptuous. Yes, clothes hang better on thinner bodies, but naked bodies look sexier with curves. While women worry about how their clothes look and what the scales say, men are visualising the body underneath. Scarlett Johansson always ranks high in the sexiest women in the world lists, but Alexa Chung is idolised by the fashionistas. That high-fashion Alexa body, all ribs and hips without an ounce of flab, probably works better dressed than undressed.

And there is a problem with the eroticisation of eating, as exemplified by female TV chefs like Nigella, Sophie Dahl, Rachel Khoo etc. We all know that Nigella's TV presence is about 10 per cent recipes, and 90 per cent kitchen porn! The food looks delicious, of course, but really it's about the finger-licking and flirtatious glances to camera; the televisual equivalent of chocolate body-paint. Nigella's body is far from 'perfect' but her lascivious mix of cooking and curves is the perfect male fantasy: food and sex miraculously rolled into one.

Men love Nigella, of course. They may say that women should eat more; they may enjoy the waitress-in-a-diner fantasy, or the showgirl, or the buxom milking maid; they may be turned on by girls who eat burgers and milkshakes and messy (sexy) food. The hearty appetite promises sexual rapaciousness. It's true, a hungry woman toying with her salad is anti-social and depressing. But how else are we supposed to stay slim?

This is where the 'female celebrity with a huge appetite' routine comes from. Known as DIPE (Documented Instance of Public Eating) it's the charade whereby skinny actresses and models tuck into a full English breakfast in front of the interviewer to emphasise their normal, healthy love of food. It doesn't have to be a full English – a roast dinner, or hamburger, or generous helping of pasta does just as well. Look at me, they seem to say, I'm slender and beautiful *and boy can I eat*! Of course this is a finely constructed piece of image-crafting (because the rest of the time they're existing on wheatgrass shots and cigarettes). And this is why so many of us 'civilians' feel betrayed by our own bodies: our chocolate cravings and our lardy bits.

If being on a diet is unsexy, then is being overweight sexy? To put it another way, how do you become one of these women who can eat anything she wants, all voracious and insatiable, and still have an uber-body? Plenty of us weigh the same as Scarlett, Nigella or Kelly, but our curves aren't in the same places. They pour it all into this smoulderingly-sexy, to-die-for silhouette, and we feel completely inadequate by comparison. Pasty and flabby and fat.

A. A. Gill's comments are a reminder that women can't win, and a slap in the face for anyone who has ever tried to lose weight to attract the opposite sex:

'The worst look on a women is a diet. The best? Fish and chips.'

*

What do fish and chips have to do with it?

Sex and food are two of the most loaded issues of our time. Both are natural human instincts and yet both are often associated with shame and secrecy. It cannot be a coincidence that most eating disorders surface during puberty, a time of rapid emotional and physical development. As teenagers our appetites for food and sex increase: our growing bodies demand both. In Western societies, food and sex are everywhere, and yet we have a confused relationship with both. Like food, sex and sexual images are highly visible – in magazines and on TV, on the high street and the Internet. Food and sex are simultaneously universal and forbidden; sources of deep pleasure and intense guilt.

We use similar terms to refer to both food and sex: *temptation, satisfaction, craving, giving in*. We tell young people – women especially – to eat healthily and fully, to explore their bodies and embrace their sexuality – and yet everywhere we worship diets, slimming, and sexual fidelity. We don't practise what we preach, and it's hard to know what we're even preaching: the messages about bodies and appetites, self-respect and sex are horribly conflicted.

I think the link between the two hungers is particularly acute for women. We are supposed to be highly sexual, in touch with our own bodies, having multiple orgasms, with our impeccable Brazilian waxes, and the perfect man. We should be liberated enough to have one-night stands (but really, nice girls don't). We should be laddish enough to eat burgers with the boys; we should love our bodies *just as we are*, while also looking amazing in a bikini. It may sound a little 'third wave' to admit this, but the female body is currency.

Many women experience this overload of desire and hunger; the need for control while feeling out of control. Yearning, frustration and sexual pleasure, intense cravings for carbs, sugar or fat (often triggered by dieting) are not so very different. Moderation is hard. Resorting instead to extremes – alcohol, food or sex – can be a desperate attempt to fill up the gaping hole inside. Eating disorders often develop as a response to feeling out of control in other areas: the bingeing and purging of bulimia in particular are a desperate all-or-nothing attitude to one's own body.

I emailed my friend C to ask about her bulimia at Oxford. She replied: 'We'd spend all day drinking in the pub, remember? When we got back I'd eat and eat, toast and cereal, all the crisps and biscuits in my cupboards, all the leftovers in the fridge.' At the time, deep in anorexia, I didn't even know she had an eating disorder. Her email ends: 'Thinking back, it's frightening to realise how violent it was – I really despised myself. Stuffing myself and then vomiting was a frenzy of self-hatred.'

In *Eating, Drinking, Overthinking* the psychologist Susan Nolen-Hoeksema describes these excesses as the 'toxic triangle' which can push women over the edge: 'Whereas men tend to externalise stress – blaming other people for their negative feelings or difficult circumstances – women tend to internalise it, holding it in their bodies and minds.'

When pain is internalised in this way, it can trigger worse problems. Some academic studies claim that up to 80 per cent of patients with eating disorders also have a history of abuse. The links between eating disorders and sexual assault make sense – something about punishing oneself, denying one's own needs, the betrayal of the body, finding a focus for the shame/hurt. Sexual abuse makes them feel intensely guilty, as does food hunger, so they try to deny themselves everything. Victims of sexual abuse often blame themselves, thinking that they must have invited the abuse: they cannot control or punish the offender so they damage their own bodies and punish themselves. The parallels between sexual abuse and disordered eating are logical, when you think about the self-hatred caused by both conditions. (I should say, this hasn't been my experience, nor that of many women I know with EDs, but it's thought-provoking nonetheless.)

It's a vicious circle of course: natural human needs cannot be managed by abstinence or excess, and the more you deny yourself, the more you crave. As someone who got caught up for so long in the cycle of starvation, I think it's about learning to trust oneself. Anorexia isn't about being thin so much as it is about *control*. I felt that if I started to eat, I would never be able to stop – so it was safer not to start at all. It is illogical but you can see my reasoning.

I had lost that most basic gift: trusting oneself. I'm not religious, and I never felt guilty about sex. But I did (and sometimes still do) feel guilty about eating.

We all need food, and most of us enjoy sex: there is no point in feeling bad about either of these appetites. The trick is to find a balance, which can be surprisingly hard. Compulsive eating, purging, being sexually promiscuous, starving or binge-drinking: these all come from a place of inner emptiness; a misdirected attempt to fill the void. They're destructive and addictive, and they lead you back to the place where you started: self-loathing.

*

A 2011 survey found that 51 per cent of women would give up sex for a year if it meant they could be skinny. Of the 2,500 women surveyed by US *Fitness* magazine, over half said they would choose 'the body of their dreams' instead of sex, while the other 49 per cent said they would rather have great sex and be 15 kg overweight.

Great sex. What does that mean nowadays? It used to mean being with someone attractive who cared about you, who wanted to connect on a physical level, to be emotionally open and sexually aware (but without being clingy or feeble; no Sting-style tantric sex sessions please). In other words, a man who understood a little about the female body, and was willing to put the time in to make sex good for you as well as for himself. These days that all sounds a bit *Joy of Sex*, doesn't it? These days it's about being as wild as possible, and ideally tweeting the sex-tapes afterwards. According to Naomi Wolf, anal fissures are now among the top sexual health concerns of young women. How sad is that?

Along with the general pornification of women's bodies (and food) the sexual act seems to have become a competitive sport.

Another arena in which women have to excel; another activity in which they are being judged. When I was seventeen, discussing with school-friends about when and how we would lose our virginity, there was a dim awareness of pornography; that our boyfriends and brothers passed smutty copies of *Playboy* around the playground. I don't think we discussed positions or techniques (although I do remember one of the cool girls talking about 'what to do when he's going down on you'. The solution, apparently, was to light a cigarette!).

But we didn't expect to be compared to the centrefold women in porn mags, with their legs splayed in that curiously repulsive pose. We never felt the need to look anything like a *Playboy* bunny. The expectation – and the reality – was that seeing their girlfriend's naked body, no matter how imperfect, would be a delight and a dream come true for any seventeen-year-old male. Teenage boys now have easy access to pornography online where female bodies are more surgically modified than ever before. As discussed in the Ministry of Gym, the Internet sex industry is a growing problem, with boys as young as seven being exposed to explicit and often violent sexual acts online.

As the demands on normal women to look like porn stars increase, the emphasis on female pleasure seems to have diminished. It's more important to look a certain way in bed, to be 'adventurous' (in other words, hardcore) than it is to be in a mutually satisfying sexual relationship. We all know the statistics about how many women fake orgasms (from 50–75 per cent, depending on who you believe); we all know that it requires time and trust and patience to reach that level of female arousal. How much harder it must be to relax and enjoy yourself when you're up against the plastic perfection of Internet porn. Great sex doesn't look or sound perfect. Whatever E. L. James claims, it's rare to 'climax' when engaged in the anxious task of losing your virginity.

Ah yes, Anastasia… She and Christian Grey have a lot to answer for. In 2012, the publishing sensation that is *Fifty Shades of Grey* (and its myriad spin-offs) brought hardcore sex into the open in the oddest way. Reading the book – in order to write a review for a national newspaper I hasten to add – I was shocked at the nastiness of it all. I didn't feel aroused in the slightest. I hated it. The sex is, frankly, embarrassing: all that gasping and role play and grasping of erections. These were not fantasies I had secretly harboured; I didn't want Christian Grey to turn up at my door and dominate me as he dominates Anastasia.

I'm not repressed: I understand the theme of sexual power-play; the thrill of being slightly dominant, or slightly submissive, of course. Books, films and private fantasies are erotic, surely, because they tap into something raw and human within us. You do and say things in bed which you wouldn't say in broad daylight (usually). But the sex in *Fifty Shades* simply isn't erotic – it wears itself out with endless repetition – and the writing is worse than Mills and Boon.

Our heroine Anastasia starts out as a virginal twenty-two-year-old and quickly becomes an accomplished sex goddess. She is every man's wet dream: a deep-throat champion who loves to swallow, voracious in bed, and multi-orgasmic to boot. She is overcome by Christian's power and manliness – he is her dominant, her master, a man who holds his erection in his hand and introduces it thus: 'I want you to become well acquainted, on first-name terms if you will, with my favourite and most cherished part of my body.' I think the whole point of the book is its kinkiness – it can't be its storyline – but how is this kinky? *Lady Chatterley's Lover* is fifty times kinkier.

So, the sex in *Fifty Shades* didn't do it for me. What else? The only element which I found vaguely noteworthy was the role of food in relation to sex; Anastasia claims never to be hungry (even after marathon sex sessions) but then gorges on junk food with her best friend. A constant theme of the book is how she's super thin and can't put on any weight. Christian is endlessly trying to force her to eat: 'Of course you'll have something to eat,' he snaps. 'Pancakes, bacon and eggs.' 'Eat what's on your plate.' Quelle coincidence that the heroine's name can be shortened to Ana...

'CONTRACT APPENDIX ONE. *The submissive will eat regularly to maintain her health and wellbeing.*' This is one of the clauses of a sexual contract the 'dominant' Christian Grey wants Anastasia to sign – something that women in real S/D relationships have seen as laughable at best.

'"We know what we want." Christian's mouth twitches with a small, sexy smile. "Two portions of buttermilk pancakes with maple syrup and bacon on the side, and two glasses of orange juice."'

There is plenty of speculation online about Anastasia and her attitude to food, most of them starting, 'Is it just me, or has anyone else detected eating disorders in *Fifty Shades*...' Christian tells Ana he has 'issues with wasted food'. Whatever the message about eating and sex – confused, at best – there's no doubt that both characters have issues with food. I know I'm not the only who finds this million-selling bonkbuster book a load of crap.

*

The interaction between sex and food – the interplay between female restraint and pleasure – can be acutely complex. Even without all the diet, weight and body-shape issues, there is a sense that women should keep themselves under control, while also letting go. As we've seen, it's sexy to eat, but not sexy to be fat.

In a similar way, the relationship between appearance and attraction is complicated. While there is a consensus among the media on what perfection looks like (bland, blonde, young), in real life it's impossible to generalise. Men, like women, want different things – and usually we want what we don't have. Very thin women often talk about being unable to gain weight, and longing for curves; fat women would love to feel boyish, or to go without a bra.

My mother had a bizarre, but touching, encounter in her local Oxfam shop the other day. She was trying on a black 1920s-style flapper dress, all feather and sequins, and stepped out of the changing room to look in the full-length mirror. As she stood there, a middle-aged man approached her and asked for a quick cuddle.

'A cuddle?' she asked warily... 'um, do we know each other?' He explained that he had been married to a fat woman for twenty years and – 'I just wanted to hold a slim woman in my arms.' She politely explained that her husband was waiting for her outside the shop.

It can be surprising to discover who and what we find attractive. Many of us talk about having a 'type' but in reality it's just a fiction: you may think you go for tall, dark men and end up with a short chap with ginger hair. How often do we find ourselves falling for people gradually, as we get to know them: friends, colleagues, people we spend time around and grow towards. I've met handsome men who I'm not remotely attracted to; I've fallen head-over-heels in lust with slightly geeky, or balding, or greying men. One of the most devastating relationships of my life was with someone who, objectively speaking, now has a paunch and not much hair left. And yet for many years I would have walked over hot coals for that man. For me, there is no automatic association between good looks and sexual chemistry. Is it lame to admit that I find bad spelling a turn-off? (I once broke up with a man because he held his pen in his fist, like a harpoon. In love letters he would misspell 'you're' as 'your'; imagine: 'your so beautiful'.)

Sex appeal isn't simple. It's not simple from the inside either, when you're the one gaining or losing weight. Getting the perfect body doesn't give you the perfect life. My anorexia was sparked by various factors (broken heart, diet gone wrong, faulty brain chemistry) but it was never about getting the perfect body. I attracted more male interest at my highest weight than at my lowest weight. As I dropped pounds, and then stones, I didn't flaunt my body; soon I was actively hiding it. In general, very thin women don't flaunt it. There might have been a few months when I looked great – some tipping point between nine and a half stone and five a half stone, when I felt super-slim and sexy. I don't remember it. I was sliding so fast.

I do remember one Friday night, when the man who was at the root of it all casually turned up in Oxford (as you do, just passing through from New York City). Of course I let him in; of course we drank two bottles of wine; of course we ended up in bed. During the course of that weekend, as he held me in his arms, a bundle of bones, he kept asking what had happened. How had I turned from the glowing nineteen-year-old who kissed him goodbye in Manhattan to this skeletal twenty-one-year-old?

What could I say? *Losing you is eating me up from the inside; I am completely worthless without you...* If I couldn't have him, it seems, I was going to deny myself everything, food included. To me, thin has never felt sexy. It turns out Wallis Simpson was wrong: you can be too thin.

Chapter 8

THE MINISTRY OF SURGERY

Once the Ministries of Beauty and Diet have convinced you of your shortcomings as a woman, it's time to make an appointment with the men in white coats. Welcome to the Ministry of Surgery, a world of private consultations and pain, where scalpels and cannulas will slice and suck away your imperfections. It's a magic universe where injections will freeze your muscles and eliminate your wrinkles and inflate your thin lips. In the months to come, you'll look at those before and after photographs and realise just how wrong you were before and how perfect you are now. Right?

As the range of cosmetic surgery grows, the list of physical flaws increases. Logically speaking, our noses, breasts or vaginas should be no uglier than they were one hundred years ago. But, under intense pressure from the media and advertising industries, we absorb the images of other, more perfect women and begin to believe that our bodies are indeed saggy, protuberant, shameful.

Just as we know that everything will be better when we're thinner, so we realise that life would be better if only we were smoother, tighter, smaller. We stare into the mirror and back at the magazines; we compare ourselves with digitally enhanced images of the female body, and feel all wrong.

But surely, the argument goes, cosmetic surgery empowers us as women, giving us the bodies we always dreamed of? No. It's not empowering, and it's not about reshaping or refining: it's violence dressed up as choice. Cosmetic surgery invites us to enter a dystopian universe in which everybody looks the same: poreless, ageless, blonde and bland. And it's a hugely powerful, billion-dollar industry dedicated to wholly unnecessary operations to sculpt women's bodies into the form they take in male teenage fantasies, or porn films, or airbrushed advertisements. The re-sculpting is often unsuccessful, and then you're on the scrap-heap anyway. How did we reach the stage where female bodies are treated as commodities? We are sentient beings, not things. Women's magazines routinely refer to body MOTs as if we were cars or machines, to be waxed and re-sprayed, and when we get old and rusty, to be given an overhaul.

The term 'cosmetic' is intentionally misleading: look at the brutality of these procedures. Why are women paying thousands of pounds to men (and they are mostly men) in surgical masks to have their noses broken, their cheekbones sawn down, their jaws clamped and stomachs stapled, their eyelids sliced and hairlines lifted? Have you seen the bleeding and the bruising, have you read about the fluid loss, the skin ulceration and infection, the nerve paralysis? I don't think there's anything sadder than those stretched, painful, frozen expressions. Scalpels and Botox – cutting and poison. How did it get so bad for women?

(Of course it's important to acknowledge that growing numbers of men are having cosmetic surgery, a worrying trend which reflects the increase in male eating disorders and body dysmorphia. But overwhelmingly it is still women going under the knife or the needle: around 90 per cent of procedures are carried out on women, so I will refer to women in this chapter – with apologies to our brothers-in-arms.)

In general, I'm all for choice. If a diet or an exercise regime makes you feel healthier and more confident, go for it. If, in extreme cases, a physical abnormality is causing psychological distress, cosmetic surgery can be a positive solution. Similarly after an accident or other disfigurement, reconstructive surgery is a wonderful thing. But most women aren't having it for these reasons. They're undergoing unnecessary operations because they have been made to feel there is something wrong with the way they are.

Back in 1990 Naomi Wolf wrote in *The Beauty Myth* that women who underwent surgery were fighting to stay loved, relevant, employed, admired; they were fighting against time running out. Less than twenty-five years later the situation is much worse. Surgery is now carried out on women of all ages, and almost anything is available. It's gone way beyond anti-ageing surgery for older women: teenage and young women are bombarded with dishonest digital images of how the perfect female should look. For women, the body has become a source of intense anxiety.

Whether it's classed as surgical or non-surgical treatment, knives or injections, there is something deeply disturbing about the new uniform beauty; the notion that our body parts should be a certain size and shape, and never show signs of gravity, personality or age.

*

According to Simon Cowell, Botox is 'no more unusual than toothpaste'. While Botox is certainly becoming more popular, for most of us civilians there is still quite a gulf between the two.

Botulinum toxin is a protein and neurotoxin produced by the bacterium *Clostridium botulinum*. This lethal, naturally occurring substance can cause botulism, a serious and life-threatening illness in both humans and animals. Botulinum toxin has also been recognised as a potential weapon of bioterrorism.

Scientists have been researching the therapeutic use of Botulinum toxin for decades. In the 1950s they discovered that injecting overactive muscles with minute quantities of the toxin helped alleviate the eye conditions blepharospasm and strabismus, chronic migraines and cerebral palsy, and excessive sweating. Injected into expression lines, and to prevent the creases caused by frowning, scowling, smiling or looking surprised, Botox works by blocking the nerve impulses that tell a muscle to contract. The amount of Botox injected determines how much expression you have. More Botox means less expression. The three most common areas for Botox injections are in the forehead, around the 'crow's feet' area of the eyes, and between the eyebrows (glabellar lines, or so-called 'lion's wrinkles').

And the bad news? Adverse side effects may include inappropriate facial expression such as drooping eyelids, double vision, uneven smile, or loss of the ability to close eyes, headaches, dysphagia, flu-like syndromes, blurred vision, dry mouth, fatigue, allergic reactions and swelling or redness at the injection site.

The global Botox market is forecast to reach $2.9 billion by 2018. Since 2007 Botox has been the most common cosmetic operation, with nearly 5 million procedures in the United States alone. The number of women in the UK having Botox each year broke the million mark back in 2010, but it's hard to know how widespread it really is. After all, if Botox is doing its job properly, it should be invisible. The high-profile cases are well-known of course: the aforementioned Simon Cowell is a self-confessed Botulinum junkie. Many other celebrities are fans of Botox, often detectable from their limited facial expressions, as are the silicone addicts, routinely ridiculed in the media for their over-filled, pillow-lipped appearance – the so-called 'trout pout'. So strange, these forty-somethings, looking younger than their twenty-something selves.

Like other beauty treatments, cosmetic surgery is steadily infiltrating the mainstream. What used to be demanded of models and actresses is now demanded of us all: the Ministry of Surgery expects us to be baby-smooth and wrinkle-free. Cosmetic Botox, which until recently was considered fairly radical, is now available in beauty salons, dentists, spas, and even at high-street pharmacies. In March 2012 Superdrug announced it would be rolling out a chain of in-store Pro Skin clinics, offering anti-wrinkle injections, laser hair removal and microdermabrasion. Prices start at £149 for Botox – compared with around £300 for Botox in a Harley Street clinic. Superdrug is great for beauty bargains, but the notion of having Botox injections, half-price, along with your lunchtime sandwich, seems a step too far.

So do you get the magic jabs; do your friends get them? What about laser teeth-whitening? It used only to be real movie stars like Tom Cruise who had blindingly white smiles. These days laser-whitening is the first rung on the public ladder of success – one of the first things all X Factor finalists have to do is have their teeth whitened (forget their singing voices). Home-bleaching dental kits are available for as little as £19.99 online.

We have witnessed the creeping normalisation of other cosmetic operations too. Facelifts used to be the preserve of eccentric old Hollywood has-beens, but these days mainstream female newsreaders are open about their facelifts at the age of forty or fifty; TV presenters discuss their gastric bypasses on-air; and breast implants and liposuction are *de rigueur*. Botox is increasingly seen as routine in the anti-ageing war, almost as normal as dyeing your hair to conceal the perfidious grey streaks. You don't even need to be middle-aged to benefit: many surgeons recommend that Botox should start as early as our twenties so that facial lines do not have the chance to form. Pre-emptive action, if you will.

All this has been creeping up on us, I think. Partly it's the trickle-down effect: when some beautiful women are endlessly youthful and wrinkle-free we should all be, shouldn't we? Then there's the intense media scrutiny and the stream of Internet images of female perfection. TV and film are now in High Definition, which is unforgiving of any signs of decrepitude or facial expression. The advertising industry also encourages us to feel ashamed of ageing, and to regard it as a choice: we don't have to look like wrinkled hags; if only we would buy more of their miracle products we could 'turn back the clock'. This is one situation where it would be nice to feel less responsible: because we're not responsible for ageing really. Beyond eating healthily, not smoking, and not sunbathing, there isn't much you can do about it. And most of us know that cosmetic surgery, however skilfully performed, isn't really the solution.

*

'Let's do breakfast, darling...' I recently met up with my friend V at Villandry in Great Portland Street. A stone's throw from Harley Street and the Portland Women's Hospital, it's a delicious cafe, restaurant and delicatessen (and a favourite haunt of the wealthy and cosmetically enhanced). V is nearly 50, a motivational speaker, homeopath, and former singer in a band. She is a hilarious mix of hippy chick and image-conscious business-woman and I adore her: she has an all-year-round suntan and perfect highlights, she wears her aviator sunglasses even in winter; she fiddles with various silver phones and the keys of her Audi, and she does that thing of glancing over your shoulder to see if any more important people are nearby.

From talking about food, to relationships, love and heartbreak, we got onto the subject of ageing. It transpired that she'd been having regular Botox injections since the age of thirty-five. Here's where it got tricky. According to V, because she started Botox so early, she still retains the youthful looks of her thirties: 'On a good day I'd say I look thirty-five,' she says. But she doesn't: Botox doesn't make her look younger, just smoother. Botox may stop you from scowling or frowning but it doesn't prevent the formation of fine lines and wrinkles, however young you start. V still looks like a woman in her late forties: incredibly well-preserved and expensively high-maintenance, but not thirty-five. You can't literally turn back the clock.

But I came away from that meeting feeling quite anxious. It was just before I started filming for Channel 4, and I was already worrying about how I came across on-screen. It's one thing to be tagged in a dodgy photo on someone's Facebook page – but on television, in front of 3.1 million viewers? I find I don't have the usual female hang-ups about my weight or body-shape (ironic, I know) but I hate looking old. From what V said, practically every other female TV presenter my age is well into their Botox. If they're all perfectly fresh-faced and line-free, then how ancient am I going to look?

And yet I won't do it. I refuse to go there. I'm sure it would be miraculously rejuvenating, and very addictive. I can't afford a beauty habit that pricey (although the cost of Botox will doubtless continue to fall as it becomes increasingly mass-market). I'll admit that I considered it: maybe just a few jabs, before we started filming? To look nice on camera in HD?

It's like getting highlights, but worse. After an adolescence spent creating personal hair-disasters with Sun-In (anyone who grew up in the 1990s will know what I mean) in my twenties I started getting my blonde highlights done professionally. It costs a bomb, and of course it's never-ending, because the roots grow out, and the whole process starts again. And that's how I think about Botox: the effects usually last three to six months, gradually wearing off, and then you have to repeat it. The everyday maintenance of being a woman – what my little sister and I refer to as the 'shaving and plucking and cropping and weeding' – is tedious enough. I don't think I can cope with adding Botox to that list of regular ugly-fighting upkeep.

Also, what's the point? Time and expense and moral outrage aside, I don't think Botox works. While it freezes your muscles, and therefore makes your face move less, it doesn't make you more beautiful. To me, V's forehead looks odd: suspiciously smooth and tight. The rest of her body is visibly 49 years old – the usual veins on her hands and forearms, slacker skin on her neck – but her face is weirdly line-free. Many celebrities suffer from this over-Botoxed look: plumped-up and shiny. It's not as extreme as the wind-tunnel effect of old-fashioned facelifts, but it certainly isn't natural.

A friend of mine who works as a TV runner and location assistant encounters these women close up: 'They don't see it – the way most of us don't really see how we look from the outside. They keep topping up the collagen in their lips and the fillers in their cheeks, and they can't see how weird their faces are becoming.' This is the risk, that those anti-ageing jabs, the discreet nips and tucks, become less and less subtle as the years go by.

*

Strictly speaking, Botox isn't cosmetic surgery: it is classed as non-surgical, one of the so-called 'lunchtime' procedures. Is a needle any less invasive than a scalpel; where do we draw the line? It seems important to make a distinction, but I acknowledge my own inconsistencies. I find some female 'grooming' procedures acceptable – highlights, laser hair removal, eyebrow threading – whereas Botox, fillers and implants make me mad. Maybe it depends on the degree of invasiveness: the introduction of a foreign substance into the body, be that silicone or muscle paralysers; maybe it's about the pain involved, or the cost, or the instruments.

When it comes to make-up, lotions and potions, the cosmetics industry is like an expensive world of smoke and mirrors, where intelligent consumers get hypnotised by meaningless gobbledegook about antioxidants, skin renewal, and cell boosting technologies. We want to believe the anti-ageing hype, or we want to buy ourselves a treat, so we suspend our usual common sense and hand over our credit cards to the women behind the beauty counters, half-aware that none of these products will take ten years off our age. As one part of our brain is saying *This miracle product will reveal my inner radiance, erase signs of fatigue, and turn back time*, the other half is saying *Really? £90 for a tube of under-eye serum? You sucker...*

The expense and the glamour is part of the deception – we know that – the French names, the faux-scientific terminology of Q10 this, and RVF-10 that, the elaborate packaging...

At what point does illusion become exploitation? Take, for example, the case of Rodial – a company who make some startling claims for transformation. According to the founder, Maria Hatzistefanis, Rodial uses 'cutting-edge science to create a range of high-tech, innovative, fast-acting and highly effective products that offer radical results without the need for surgery.'

This promise of miracle anti-ageing 'without the need for surgery' sounds almost too good to be true, as do some of their other products:

- Glamoxy Snake Serum – a neuropeptide that mimics the effects of the temple viper's potent venom to instantly lift the face
- Arm Sculpt – to banish bingo wings, containing Lipocare to stimulate fat-burning and the transformation of fat into energy
- Boob Job – a £127 breast-enlargement cream offering a non-invasive alternative to surgery and an increase of up to half a cup size after 56 days
- Tummy Tuck – which can reduce the abdominal area by up to 2 cm in eight weeks
- Crash Diet – a gel scientifically proven to help with the breakdown of stubborn fat

Boob job, tummy tuck and crash diet – larger breasts in a jar – an instant facelift – you couldn't make it up! I was recently sent a bee venom face mask from another company (which retails at £75 and made absolutely no difference to my face, except for a slight stinging sensation) but snake venom is new to me.

Many cosmetic companies refer to their 'active ingredients', one of those nebulous concepts like 'superfood' which is hard to prove or disprove. But there is no independently published scientific evidence that using a cream can make you thinner. Chris Griffiths, Professor of Dermatology at Manchester University, says that to have any effect, a cream would have to penetrate well beneath the surface of the skin into the subcutaneous fat: 'I think a lot of women who buy these products do so for the same reason men buy expensive cars – it makes them feel good.' He's right, and maybe it does us no harm. After all, there are worse things in the world than believing that a caffeine-infused cream will actually eliminate cellulite (as promised by Fat Girl Slim products) or that a mascara will make eyelashes up to twelve times longer. Maybe these expensive products are just a bit of fun for those with money to burn.

*

Beyond creams and serums, the distinction between surgical and non-surgical is becoming even hazier – with potentially grave consequences. Many politicians, health campaigners and even plastic surgeons have spoken of a 'Wild West' culture which allows GPs and dentists to perform breast enlargements and anyone to inject dermal fillers. In 2012 a leader in *The Times* declared: 'It beggars belief that dermal fillers are not classified as prescription drugs.' In this country, around 140 dermal fillers can be legally used – even in the US, home of cosmetic surgery, they are classed as medicine and only a small number are allowed.

What is it with all this acid, poison and abrasion? Along with the modern mania for detoxing, we are encouraged to scourge and purify in the most alarming way. I remember when my sisters and I were teenagers, we made one of those home-made body scrubs from a magazine – coarse sea salt in honey or olive oil or something. I ended up ripping the skin on my thighs to shreds! These days I've upgraded to a posh all-natural body brush, although I don't often bother to use it. Over the millennia, our skin has developed a perfectly good system of self-renewal. There's actually no need for the endless exfoliation, is there?

Remember when a professional facial was a girly spa treat, something you might enjoy with your sister or best friend. These days facials have all the pampering qualities of an industrial sander, with dermabrasion and laser resurfacing among the most popular procedures. Chemical peels are another way of blasting off the top layer of your face – dead skin cells, age spots and all. The actress Jennifer Aniston recently discussed her predilection for the chemical peel: 'It's extremely intense... you look like a battered burn victim for a week. The dead skin on your face just kind of falls off, for eight days.'

If that's not grim enough, what about a Vampire Facial? Platelet Rich Plasma (PRP) therapy, also known as the Vampire Facelift, is a procedure that entails having blood drawn from your arm. The extracted blood is spun in a centrifuge to separate out the platelets and then injected back into the wrinkles in your face, in order to stimulate new collagen production. Really.

On his own website, American dermatologist Troy Thompson explains: 'Shortly after the treatment [patients] begin to see a baby soft fresh skin with an immediate change in skin texture, wrinkles, fine lines and pigmentation – with a collagen renewal that continues for up to five months after the procedure.'

The actress Anna Friel has admitted to being a fan of the Vampire Facial: 'It's like they take your blood and they mix it up and separate it, it's really scientific and natural but it makes a difference.' She said she couldn't do what she called 'the freeze' (Botox injections) because 'as an actress my face has to move'. She also likes Cryoderm facials, costing around £500 a pop, before her red-carpet appearances. Why should a beautiful actress – or any woman for that matter – feel the need to undergo such bizarre treatments in order to enhance their looks?

*

Take a good look in the mirror: how badly do you score against the latest invented face-crimes? Depending on your age, you may or may not have some of the following: lines around the mouth – or perorial wrinkles; creases running from nose to mouth – or naso-labial furrows; laughter lines around the eyes – or crow's feet (for which there is Crowtox, special Botox for crow's feet); pigmentation and spider veins and age spots. Every blemish is a permanent reminder of your former sunbathing crimes, or smoking crimes, or smiling crimes. As teenagers we longed for hormonal breakouts/acne to end; and yet ageing skin makes adolescent skin seem idyllic by comparison.

The newest invented sin with which to frighten us is *rides du lion* (those glabellar lines, or lion's wrinkles). These tiny vertical wrinkles on the forehead, on the small patch of skin between the eyebrows, arrived from France in 2012. I was half-outraged, half-resigned when I first heard about lion's wrinkles – I suppose like many women I've given up feeling surprised at the bullshit directed at us. I covered this in my *Times* column that week, as did several female journalists in other papers. Faced with such ludicrous body-fascism, what can you do but smile. I enjoyed the vigorous responses at *The Guardian* online:

- How in the name of all that's holy have we allowed things to go this far? It's outrageous to think there are vast swathes of human beings out there consumed by self-loathing when all that's happening is the natural process of ageing. Alright some of us do it better than others but whatever you try and however much money you spend you won't stop it. More importantly, getting old is not a crime.

- We age and it's tough but there it is. It's a fact of life.

- Why should we allow ourselves to feel a failure because things are beginning to sag a bit? There's nothing wrong with making the best of what you've got... but please don't sit down in front of the mirror filling your wrinkles from a tube every day and then worry about the wretched stuff peeling off if you have a menopausal flush. By all means, luxuriate in a new moisturiser, slather on a new body cream or try the latest lash lengthening mascara – all these things are wonderful mood lifters. But please, PLEASE, don't fall for the hype.

And that's just above the neck — for our bodies we have a cruel vocabulary with which to lacerate ourselves: bingo wings, cankles and muffin tops. Cellulite is a shameful failing, while saggy upper arms should be kept out of sight. Stomachs that have carried babies, breasts that have suckled them, have 'unsightly' stretch marks. Decolletages (crepey?); buttocks and knees (drooping?); vagina (too loose?). No female body part escapes the scrutiny of the men in white coats, the self-hatred and the surgical correction. The language of disgust would be funny if it wasn't so depressing – it's no wonder that atelophobia, the fear of imperfection, is on the increase.

What I most object to is the fear and the shame, this sense that we have so much to cover up. Think, for a moment, of how your boyfriend, husband, male friend or brother looks when he wakes up in the morning. Into the shower, brush teeth and shave, then dress and breakfast. Wash and go, right? Then compare that with the exfoliating and conditioning, the styling and blow-drying of hair, the cleansing and toning and making-up, the tights, high heels and handbags. Leave aside menstruating, being pregnant, giving birth, or other optional extras, just being female is a time-consuming business. Imagine not doing anything to your appearance for six weeks. I don't just mean not applying cosmetics, I mean no razors or tweezers or hair-dye; no treatments, nothing to conceal the way your appearance naturally is. Just washing and going. Would that be OK – are you OK with the real you?

I would find it hard, I admit. There have been times when I've not had time or access to decent lighting/bathrooms – and it's amazing how quickly everything falls apart. On a recent road trip across America I remember I hadn't bothered to pluck my eyebrows for a couple of weeks: by the time we rolled into another state, another hotel room each evening, I was too exhausted to bother with 'upkeep'. I remember how Neanderthal (I felt) I looked, arriving back in the UK, all sprouty and a bit wild! And yet there must be a sensible level at which we can say: thus far and no more. No needles, perhaps; no scalpels? I fear the current spread of cosmetic surgery, because coercion may be close behind. Once things are accepted, they quickly become expected. Like other aspects of female appearance, it's a kind of mission creep. The higher the bar, the harder we must toil to change the way we look naturally. Already the expectations are abhorrent: that women will be virtually hairless, for example. Soon we'll all have to wear false nails and hair extensions, our make-up will be tattooed on, and no one will dare to go grey. There was nothing wrong with the way we looked before, but the new normal spreads and spreads.

*

Around the world, more than 17 million cosmetic surgery procedures take place every year. The US tops the list with 3.03 million operations; followed by Brazil's 2.4 million, China's 2.19 million, India's 0.89 million and Mexico's 0.83 million. The UK comes eighteenth in world rankings. As I mentioned, the vast majority of cosmetic procedures – around 90 per cent – are still carried out on women, but there has been steady growth in operations on men too, with 21 per cent growth since 2009.

The top five cosmetic surgeries for women in the UK are: breast augmentation (accounting for 25 per cent of all surgery), followed by blepharoplasty (eyelid surgery), breast reduction, face/neck lift, tummy tuck. For men, the top five surgeries are: rhinoplasty (nose), blepharoplasty, breast reduction, otoplasty (ear) and liposuction.

In 2009, the International Society of Aesthetic Plastic Surgery carried out a study of the most-requested celebrity traits, to find out how women view the perfect body. The following were rated as the most desirable:

- Lips: Angelina Jolie's pout was the most sought-after, with Julia Roberts in second place.
- Nose: Nicole Kidman was the favourite celebrity nose, with Julia Roberts in second again.
- Abdomen: Model Gisele Bundchen had the most desired midriff followed by Shakira and Demi Moore.
- Breasts: Most women wanted a bust like Pamela Anderson or Britney Spears. Interestingly, Pamela Anderson was also first on the list of what women didn't want their breasts to look like. Dolly Parton and Victoria Beckham were also on the 'not-so-hot' list of breasts.
- Buttocks: Jennifer Lopez's buttocks came top, with other choices including Halle Berry and Sandra Bullock.
- Legs: Despite being in her seventies, Tina Turner beat Cameron Diaz and Sharon Stone for the most-desired legs.

(Source: www.mya.co.uk/facts-from-figures)

Men coveted George Clooney and Brad Pitt's chin, nose and abdomen, Arnold Schwarzenegger's chest and David Beckham's legs.

Deconstructed like this – the perfect nose, chin or breast – it can be easy to forget that these are human bodies we're talking about. These are parts of a real flesh-and-blood person, not items on a shopping list. They are the inherited quirks that make you *you* – your mother's wonky nose, your father's large ears. When you start to alter what you are, where do you stop?

I've seen, at close hand, what can happen when you fixate over and then surgically adjust each bit of your body. When I left university, my first job was in a London advertising agency. Our division had a secretary called Hayley, a pretty blonde woman in her late twenties, who would book meeting rooms, arrange taxis, sort out malfunctioning photocopiers, the usual. At Easter she took two weeks off, and returned to work with a large bandage across the middle of her face. She'd had a nose job. (I was shocked – I didn't know anyone who'd had real cosmetic surgery.)

The bandage came off, and the swelling and bruising went down; her nose was smaller, neater, but her face had lost something: its distinctive, slightly horsey, Hayley-ness. She went on to have her breasts enlarged, her brow 'lifted', and some 'excess' skin on her chin and neck removed. When I last saw her, about a year ago, she looked completely different from the attractive, mischievous woman I'd first met. Now in her late thirties, her face is frozen, sad and immobile. Everything has been tweaked at different times, and none of it seems to hang together.

Have you seen Jocelyn Wildenstein? (If not, google her.) She is a rich American socialite with an extreme addiction to plastic surgery, spending an estimated 4 million dollars on modifying her face to look more 'feline'. She has been renamed the 'Bride of Wildenstein' and treated like a modern-day 'freak' by the tabloids, but her unusual appearance surely masks real psychological distress.

*

Like Botox, cosmetic surgery isn't a one-off – more of a revolving door. The NHS estimates that around 30 per cent of women who have breast augmentation will need more surgery within ten years. In theory, anyone considering surgery should be given a psychological assessment, and some access to counselling before and after the procedure. The reality is somewhat different: the British Association for Aesthetic Plastic Surgeons report that fewer than 35 per cent of clinics conduct routine psychological screening before surgery. First and foremost, surgery is a financial transaction for the clinic, and the business model is to sell as much as possible. Indeed patients often find themselves being advised on other ways they could improve their looks – with surgeons suggesting extra nips and tucks. Can you imagine a more vulnerable experience, already feeling deeply insecure, sitting in a starkly-lit consulting room, having a surgeon examining your body, highlighting the extra physical flaws you hadn't noticed, and then offering you the miracle fix? It would take a strong will not to agree.

Sir Bruce Keogh (Medical Director of the National Health Service) cited 'some pretty hard sales techniques out there. For example, some surgical interventions being offered where if you decide to have it quickly, you get a discount. I think that's scandalous. I don't think it's right that cosmetic interventions should be offered in raffles... The two-for-one offers, the introduce-a-friend, seem to me to be part of a sales technique which preys on the social vulnerability or social insecurity of people.'

As with any other commodity there are always cheaper offers and unscrupulous practitioners. It seems astonishing that anyone would go bargain-hunting for major surgery, but they do (just as they buy cut-price Botox) and the results are not always pretty. Internet forums are full of accounts of cosmetic procedures gone wrong: capsular contraction, when scar tissue around an implant shrinks, ruptures and leaks, scarring, creasing or build-up of fluid.

The journal *Obesity* has published research suggesting that patients who have liposuction can expect to see the removed fat return within a year of surgery. Fatty deposits often reappear in weird places – on the shoulders or back for example. And even when surgery goes perfectly, you can't avoid gravity. When one body part is tweaked, everything else will continue to age, downwards. Facelift patients find that tauter cheeks or eyelids begin to look strange over the years (just like my friend Hayley) as everything else shifts.

A recent *Sunday Telegraph* article quotes the surgeon Nick Percival at Cosmetic Surgery Partners: 'I always say: here is an implant of the size you want. See how heavy it is. That is going to have the long-term effect of stretching your breast.' He applies a similar warning to facelifts: 'The day after you've had your lift, gravity is pushing you down to the ground and soft tissues will be vulnerable to that pressure.'

The *Sunday Telegraph* article quotes a woman whose breast implants have hardened, ruptured and leaked silicone into her body, another woman who has undergone three facelifts in the last twenty years, and yet another whose tummy tuck and liposuction left the 'apron of skin' on her stomach looking worse than it did pre-surgery: 'It sounds strange but the area now looks older than the rest of my body. The skin is discoloured where I was cut, and it's bloated. I think the lipo in combination with the tuck has caused fatty deposits on my hips.'

The term 'cosmetic' is misleadingly lightweight for what can often be quite major surgery (doubtless that's the intention). In women's magazines, UK clinics such as Harley Medical Group and Transform portray surgery as a breezy lifestyle choice, an empowering step towards happiness and wellbeing. Young models peddling breast augmentation are pictured in strappy tops, beaming at readers in a joyful attitude of body confidence. As the woman with the tummy tuck comments: 'People go into surgery too lightly. They see supermodels with nothing bouncing up and down and they think: if I do this, I'll be happy.'

She's right: glossy advertising makes cosmetic surgery look beautiful. It sidesteps the underlying psychological ramifications of severe body dysmorphia, which may or may not be resolved by an operation. A 2011 study in the journal *Current Psychiatry Reports* found that women who underwent plastic surgery were more likely to commit suicide than those who had never tried it. Even taking out the suicides, the study found cosmetic surgery patients had a three times higher risk of death due to self-destructive behaviour such a drug-taking, binge-drinking and dangerous driving. Of course this doesn't mean that cosmetic surgery makes you suicidal – simply that it doesn't make pre-existing problems go away, and may even exacerbate them.

And yet demand is increasing year on year: despite the recession, over 43,000 surgical procedures were carried out in the UK in 2011 by members of the British Association of Plastic Surgeons (and many more carried out by non-members) compared with 10,700 procedures in 2003. However, most are relatively new surgical procedures, and we still know little about the long-term consequences. What will a woman's face repeatedly injected with Botox look like in forty years' time, I wonder?

The consequences of dodgy surgery were brought into sharp focus by the PIP scandal in the UK in late 2011. It was in March 2010 that French health regulators had discovered that the company Poly Implant Prothèse was fraudulently using non-approved industrial-grade silicone gel, intended for mattresses and rubber tubing, in its breast implants. The implants were found to carry a significant risk of rupture, potentially exposing the industrial silicone to body tissue. Surgeons across Europe were told to stop using PIP implants, the founder Jean-Claude Mas was arrested, and the company went bankrupt.

And yet the PIP story wasn't widely reported in the UK until Christmas Eve 2011. While the French Ministry of Health had been advising women to have the implants removed as a precaution, the UK Department of Health said that the evidence did not justify advising women to go through risky surgery. Breast-surgery patients appeared on TV and radio, expressing anxiety about what they really had inside their chests. Many private clinics said it was not their responsibility to remove the dodgy products because they had used them in good faith; there was confusion over the real risks, and whether the NHS should step in. Somewhere between 40,000 and 47,000 women in Britain are thought to have had the defective implants, either in the UK or at cut-price clinics in eastern and central Europe. Various health reviews were launched, and in the end it was found that the PIP implants were about twice as likely to rupture as standards models, causing women pain, swelling and discomfort.

Well before the PIP scandal – and more intensely afterwards – there have been calls to clean up the cosmetic surgery industry. For years there has been an almost total absence of regulation; even surgeons and their trade body the Independent Healthcare Advisory Services agree that the rules must be tightened up. Various reviews, committees and enquiries have been set up, and it is hoped that regulations will be introduced soon, to improve the murky and sometimes dangerous practice in the field.

Throughout the PIP episode I kept thinking *this is surreal.* Cosmetic breast implants (obviously I don't include reconstructive surgery in this category) are some kind of sick joke. Even Sir Bruce Keogh's reassurances make me shudder: 'I want to be sure that whenever you are putting something into someone, that we're quite sure of the quality of the stuff that's going in.' Women are having chicken fillets, pouches of industrial silicone, mattress fillers, whatever, inserted into their chests: but why? It seems like a sci-fi computer game – you know, where the Lara Croft characters in rubber hot pants are all thin with massive, gravity-defying boobs; some male fantasy gone wrong, or maybe it's just the general pornification of women, along with the no-body-hair policy. Why are women actually submitting to this surgery?

*

Breast implants are old hat, really – there is loads more wrong with us than just our flagging boobs. The new breed of surgery targets buttocks, calves, pectorals, even our toes and chins.

According to 2011 statistics, 20,680 chin augmentations were carried out in the US, and chin surgery has increased more than breast augmentation, Botox and liposuction combined. The most popular chin options are mentoplasty, which decreases the size of a large or jutting chin, and maxillofacial corrective surgery which actually alters the jaw position. The president of the ASPS Dr Malcolm Roth said: 'The chin and jawline are among the first areas to show signs of ageing. People are considering chin augmentation as a way to restore their youthful look just like a facelift or eyelid surgery. We know that as more people see themselves on video chat technology, they may notice that their jawline is not as sharp as they want it to be.' (Video conferencing, of all the stupid reasons to opt for surgery!)

The average cost of a chin implant in the US is $4,670; the largest UK cosmetic surgery provider, Transform, quotes a starting price of £4,290, although the procedure is still relatively rare in this country. Other increasingly popular cosmetic procedures in the US include lip augmentation (up 49 per cent), cheek implants (up 47 per cent), laser skin resurfacing (up 9 per cent), soft tissue fillers (up 7 per cent) and facelifts (up 5 per cent).

When you consider the range of cosmetic procedures the rules seem quite complex. If you were an alien, landing on Earth, you might be confused by the arbitrary nature of these rules: why should certain body parts be bigger – breasts, lips – while others should be smaller – chin, thighs? Who decides?

While we're on the subject of size, how do your genitals measure up? In another one of these seemingly random body-rules, the twenty-first century vagina must be small and neat. Never mind if it has given birth to babies, never mind if it functions fine the way it is: don't think you can get away with any imperfection.

Be honest, spread your legs. If your vagina is less than beautiful, shouldn't you be considering labiaplasty?

Yes, we have created our very own form of female genital mutilation, and it's becoming alarmingly popular. The phrase 'designer vagina' with its echoes of designer handbags or shoes used to sound like a sick misogynistic joke; now labiaplasty is offered at most cosmetic surgery clinics. Why is this? Not because female genitals have changed in the last few decades, or because women are spontaneously dissatisfied with them. No, this is a continuation of the porn-aesthetic that started in the late 1990s, when Internet porn went mainstream. Bigger is always better for the penis, and smaller is always better for the vagina. First it was the bikini wax, then the Hollywood and the Brazilian wax, then vaginal/anal bleaching, and now surgery. Male taste, as defined by the porn industry, has decreed that the vagina should look a certain way.

In 2012 more than 2,000 labiaplasty procedures were carried out on the NHS, and in the last five years there has been a fivefold increase. In 2011 the Harley Medical Group received more than 5,000 inquiries about cosmetic gynaecology, 65 per cent of them for labial reduction – where the labia are trimmed or completely removed – the rest for tightening and reshaping. The total number is likely to be much higher when considering the unregulated private sector, where thousands of operations are carried out, and where surgery costs upwards of £3,000.

Despite the increase in labiaplasty there are no universal NHS guidelines on the size and shape of normal female genitalia. Researchers say that little is known about the long-term effects of the procedure, and there is concern that patients are not receiving enough psychological support. As previously mentioned, fewer than 35 per cent of clinics carry out routine psychological screening before surgery. There is also the risk of genuine physical complications, including reduced sexual sensation, scarring, and bleeding or tearing in childbirth. When the labia are cut and restitched, they become more vulnerable to future traumas.

On the BBC News website, consultant gynaecologist Dr Sarah Creighton said her clinic sees girls as young as eleven seeking surgery. She found that although a small percentage of women do have abnormal labia that cause serious discomfort or embarrassment, in the majority of cases those with concerns had what she would consider normal-sized labia. The trend for more extreme pubic grooming leaves the labia more exposed – something which has contributed to more women seeking surgery, said Dr Creighton. One patient said: 'I thought it was going to be the end of all my problems – I thought it was going to look lovely, like a little designer vagina.' Post-surgery, the patient is still unhappy.

Scenting a profitable new area of body-paranoia, cosmetic surgeons have been falling over themselves to show women how ugly their nether regions are; to demonstrate how they can be improved upon or remediated; they promise enhanced sensitivity and increased arousal. Labiaplasty and vaginoplasty are painful, expensive, elective procedures carried out on healthy women. The euphemisms would be funny if they weren't so painful: vaginal rejuvenation (tightening), hymenoplasty (revirgination), and clitoral 'unhooding'. Pseudo-scientific terms such as 'misshapen' or 'laxity after childbirth' are bandied around, with strong judgemental overtones.

The fact is, most women never see what a normal vagina looks like, except for their own. Unless you have a female partner, or you work in healthcare, or you're exceptionally close to your friends, you rely on what genitalia look like in films or magazines, or what men seem to like. And the influence of porn on female genitals can't be overstated: it's simply more hardcore to film penetrative sex when there is no pubic hair in the way; when everything is visible. This modern obsession with the tight, hairless vagina also carries disturbingly child-like sexual associations. Vajazzling – decorating yourself with glitter and stars – is just another game of dressing up like a princess. I am not saying that all men secretly want to have sex with pre-pubescent girls, because this is certainly not the case, but there does appear to be a major problem with the mature, adult vagina.

I can't even believe I'm writing this. Is nothing private any more?

*

Perhaps this is nothing new. As early as 1906 surgeons were excising 'bag-like folds of skin' from eyelids, and performing the so-called 'mini-lift' on sagging jowls; these days it's cosmetic gynaecology. Elizabethans used to paint their faces with white lead, these days it's fake tan. We call women 'brave' when they abandon the hair dye and go grey naturally — the latest thing is young feminists deciding not to shave their armpits and blogging about it. What progress for women; how emancipated we are.

It's too simple to blame recent increases in body dysmorphia, obesity and disordered eating on the billion-dollar beauty, diet and cosmetic surgery industries, but there's no doubt that they fuel the crisis. Like Listerine a century ago, with their invention of halitosis, they perpetuate insecurities. They inform us that we're ageing 'prematurely' (a meaningless term if you think about it). They convince us at forty-five that we could/should pass for twenty-five; that we'd be happier, sexier and more youthful if only we made an effort; that, as women, our bodies are not good enough as they are.

*

In the end, of course, cosmetic surgery is an individual choice. But for this to work, it needs to be a genuine choice, not the desperate last resort of women (and men) who have been brainwashed into believing that their appearance is unacceptable. Although there are no definitive figures for all repeat procedures, the likelihood is that patients will come back for top-ups or new surgery. Put like this, it sounds rather like a drug – and many patients admit that self-tweaking is an addictive process. It's also a fantastic way of not dealing with more intractable issues. We can say 'my nose is too big so I feel ugly', rather than 'I have low-self-esteem' or 'I'm not comfortable in my skin and I simply don't know why'.

And we have to be realistic about what surgery can do: it may lift ageing flesh temporarily, but it cannot turn back time, as I saw with my friend V. It cannot resolve anything other than the physical flaw; it cannot halt gravity, or mend a broken relationship, or make you love yourself if you hate yourself. Most of us sense, deep-down, that the problem lies deeper than a roll of flab or sagging breasts.

It seems a peculiarly human trait, to focus on the negative aspects of our appearance. I remember a conversation I once had with a surgeon who told me the following story: during the First World War a psychological disorder was identified whereby injured young men became more preoccupied with their (negative) physical deficiencies than they were with their remaining (positive) physical capabilities. They began to fixate on their disabilities and injuries, and discounted the good prospects and opportunities which still remained to them. Animals don't do this. Look at a dog running along on three legs – when something goes wrong, they adapt.

The plight of the First World War soldiers reminds us that it's not just women who obsess over their perceived physical shortcomings. While writing this chapter I had a conversation with my boyfriend which made me see how even non-cosmetic surgery can become a displacement activity. About ten years ago he broke his ankle while being chased by a dog across a Greek island (long story). It was a very bad break, and ineptly treated in a series of Greek hospitals, and he's since had several operations. He doesn't limp or show any outward sign of pain – although his leg aches when he runs too far – but it's become something of a hobby-horse. He researches the latest procedures and scientific research into planing down bones, improving joints and maximising mobility. He's forever coming up with new ideas; he actually designs surgical plans which he presents to his surgeon.

He's fine now – we hardly ever talk about it. But, as he himself acknowledges, over the years his obsession has been worse when he's felt unhappy or anxious about something else. 'I sort of project everything onto the ankle – it hurts more, and I blame everything on that bad break. It's not even rational, but I think back to the time before I broke it, like I was this perfect physical specimen, and I feel so defective.'

This is how cosmetic surgery works for many patients – in reverse. They focus all their unhappiness on the perceived physical imperfection, not admitting that the underlying problem will still be there when their nose is perfectly straight.

On a wider scale, this is what so many of us do: we delay our lives, we put our happiness on hold, we tell ourselves how great everything will be when we've lost weight. The growth of unnecessary cosmetic surgery comes from the same place as the desire to be thin: a profound lack of confidence, physical and psychological insecurity, and the inability to like our bodies just the way they are.

Chapter 9

THE MINISTRY OF AGE

In Britain, women start to feel invisible at the age of forty-six.

A survey in 2011 found that once they passed their mid-forties, women began to receive fewer compliments and admiring glances from strangers, and men stopped holding doors open for them. After the age of forty-six women felt that their views and opinions were increasingly ignored, and that their male partners were ageing better than they were. Wrinkles, grey hairs and middle-age spread added to their erosion of confidence, making this a particularly difficult time for women. Nearly all the women questioned said they began struggling with their weight in their forties, and typically wanted to shed around two stone. This research was conducted by a contact lens company (Clarivu) but it hit a nerve, triggering a debate over why and how we begin to feel invisible in our later forties.

Age, like weight, is one of those near-universal issues for women: most of us would like to be slim, and most of us want to stay young – or at least young-looking. And yet, while we can do something about our weight, if we diet and exercise hard enough, there is nothing we can do about our age. Like weight, age is largely a numbers game: why should fifty make us *feel* any different from forty-nine? It's just a couple of digits – and yet it matters. Just as many of us become locked into the battle with the bathroom scales, so we dread those big birthdays: 4-0, 5-0, 6-0 and so on... Women are judged on their age, just as they're judged on their bodyweight and shape. We live in a society which idolises young and slender women: a glance in any high-end magazine shows lissom teenage models advertising handbags, shoes and cosmetics. Despite the fact that these magazines are read by, and the luxury products bought by, an older female demographic, the models are young, beautiful, and thin thin thin.

Just as men don't need to be slim to succeed, so they don't need to be young. They don't experience societal pressure to hide their age; nor are they made to feel irrelevant or marginalised simply for getting older. As women age, we spend increasing amounts of time and money concealing our own signs of ageing, dyeing grey hair, covering up wrinkles, plucking out whiskers. More and more women are turning to plastic surgery to combat the physical onslaught of time. In the end, of course, it's futile: no one can stop getting older.

That 'invisible at forty-six' survey also reported that a woman's self-esteem returns by the age of sixty (so we only have fourteen years in the wilderness). Perhaps it's our own fault; we should stop being so vain or insecure, we should just deal with the fact that we all get older, youth slips away, beauty fades. Compared to feeling exploited, or unfulfilled, or frightened, you could argue that feeling 'invisible' isn't such a big deal. But I think it is.

*

Maybe it first hits you in the changing room when you don't recognise the tired-looking woman in the mirror and then realise it's you; or the first time you walk past a construction site and can't raise a friendly leer from the builders, let alone a wolf-whistle. Recently I ran past a group of neon-jacketed young builders in my shorts and vest, and they didn't bat an eyelid. I. Felt. Invisible. Not that I want to be heckled by builders, but it's nice to be seen; to feel that people are enjoying the view. You notice when it stops. As a woman, this is what ageing means.

There is a sad irony in this. After years of worrying about our looks, of dieting and exercising to try to achieve the perfect body, of complaining of unwanted male attention or impossible standards of perfection, now we sense ourselves becoming invisible. I have talked to many female friends about this, all intelligent, confident individuals in their own right, and the experience seems to be universal. 'It shouldn't matter – I was never that reliant on men to make me feel good about myself – but since I turned fifty it's like I don't exist,' my friend S tells me. 'I feel sort of irrelevant.'

As women, this benign neglect creeps up on us. It's surprising how much we mind. And S is spot on – it's not just about male admiration. It is painful to realise that younger women don't register you, that the world in general doesn't notice you much. You don't turn heads or make any kind of impact at all. You fall off the sexual radar. You're written off, past it, menopausal; if you make a fuss about this, you're dismissed as a strident feminist or a bitter old spinster. If your children have children, suddenly you're a kindly grandmother. My mother does not allow my young nieces and nephews to call her 'Grandma' (and I don't blame her); instead they use her first name, Jean.

Of course there are women in their late forties – and late fifties for that matter – who are successful despite their age. There are many in public life, from Christine Lagarde, head of the International Monetary Fund, to Elle Macpherson, supermodel, mother and businesswoman. There are examples in our own lives:

our friends, sisters, ourselves; we no longer shrink into cardigans and curlers at the age of forty-six, as maiden aunts used to. But we live in a society which equates beauty with perfection, and perfection with youth. And that is something none of us can hang on to forever.

Is it any wonder that mature women feel invisible, surrounded by images of impossibly girlish loveliness? The veteran journalist Katharine Whitehorn (in her eighties) recently observed in her *Observer* column: 'Nowadays the older woman gets a pretty raw deal: clothes for her are shown on a bone-thin female... and ignore completely the need for covered upper arms and helpful high necks. If we're all really living longer, it's about time for some new fashions that actually do something for seniors.' Not that we need to cover our upper arms or necks, necessarily – but Whitehorn highlights the use of extremely young, thin women to sell products to more mature women. What a strange and inappropriate situation: if advertisers are targeting consumers in their forties and fifties, why not use models in their forties and fifties? Older women aren't entirely absent from TV and magazine advertising, but they tend to appear in anti-ageing beauty products (and these companies have been criticised for the high levels of airbrushing).

IVF and HRT (and countless cosmetic and surgical advances) have allowed us to blur the boundaries between late youth and early middle age, but they cannot undo time. Age may be just a number but it's also a fact. Even the most age-defying forty-six-year-old woman has to work hard to look that way.

*

And it's not only physical and sexual invisibility; women are faced with institutional invisibility too. It is a bitter pill to swallow, when you've built up your expertise in a field, to realise that success doesn't depend on your brains but on your appearance; that your visible seniority may work against you.

This is what all large corporations know but pretend not to, that men become more powerful and women less powerful, as they age. As a woman you don't win respect for your age and experience. There are a few notable exceptions of course: Angela Merkel or Theresa May are highly respected politicians, able to hold their own in a male environment; the Queen and the late Margaret Thatcher gained gravitas with the passing decades; Maggie Smith and Judi Dench are possibly the last generation of elderly actresses who look their actual age. But these women are notable because they are rare: on the whole, wrinkles and grey hairs indicate frailty and weakness. Women are made to feel they're no longer capable of doing a good job because their neck is no longer as firm or their skin as flawless.

I won't rehash the many examples of gender inequality; you see them every time you turn on the television, those silver foxes (male) with their pretty young blonde sidekicks (female). Think of Bruce Forsyth, in his mid-eighties, co-presenting *Strictly Come Dancing* with the glamorous Tess Daly: a reverse age imbalance (octogenarian woman with young male model) would be inconceivable, and comical.

Our society has decided that maturity adds gravitas to a man, no matter his appearance, weight or level of physical decrepitude. The language of ageing as applied to men – *distinguished, revered, wise, an elder statesman* – is markedly different from that of women – *menopausal, sexless, dried up, an old crone*. Ironically, it is men's sexual drive and performance which diminishes with age more often than women's. Although women make up the majority of the older population, they have long been stereotyped as lonely, frustrated and shrivelled. Compare the connotations of 'old codger' for a man, and 'old hag' for a woman. Elderly women are sometimes portrayed as physically repellent – a double whammy of ageism and sexism for us to look forward to in our twilight years.

Some random examples of powerful British chaps in the media: Jeremy Paxman, John Humphrys, Jeremy Clarkson, David Starkey, Jon Snow, Philip Schofield, Huw Edwards, Andrew Marr, John Simpson. They're not exactly box-fresh: all are well into middle-age, most are over sixty. They have grey hair and wrinkles – and some are even overweight. Can you think of ten high-profile females of the same age on television, or even five? Are any of these women fat? Do they have grey or thinning hair?

Men aren't entirely immune to the cult of youth – even male politicians are getting younger (David Cameron and Barack Obama represent this breed of youthful leader) – but there is no doubt that men in all fields remain relevant and respected well into their silver years. There was a slight kerfuffle in 2012 when the Radio 1 DJ Chris Moyles was moved aside to make way for the younger, funkier DJ Nick Grimshaw – but women have been treated this way for decades.

Female ageism began to gain prominence in 2009 when the BBC dropped Miriam O'Reilly from the television programme *Countryfile*. It became apparent that their decision to terminate her contract was based on her age, not on her TV skills: at fifty-one she was deemed too old to front a primetime programme. She subsequently won a case against them for age discrimination.

Although O'Reilly was reinstated, given a three-year contract, and briefly presented *Crimewatch*, she quit soon after. She remains outraged at the blatant gender inequality and ageism. Speaking to the *Daily Mail* she said: 'Switch on the TV any time of the day or night and you'll find plenty of middle-aged men with greying hair and wrinkles... The grotesque truth is that while older men are seen to have gravitas, older women are thought to be, if not an eyesore, then definitely a bit of a joke. You have to hunt high and low to find a woman with grey hair on TV.'

O'Reilly's use of the word 'eyesore' echoes the message being conveyed by the media, that middle-aged women are somehow unsightly. Unfortunately, television reflects the society in which we live: what we see on our screens quickly becomes the norm, whether it's *Newsnight* or *The Only Way is Essex*. When television demonstrates its contempt for older women, it makes it OK for the rest of society to do the same. Once we show the first (physical) signs of ageing, our currency as women is devalued.

O'Reilly was understandably angry at the BBC's treatment, but she is not a lone voice in the media. The newsreader Fiona Bruce has also spoken out: 'Age is definitely an issue for women in TV. I know I need to make the best of myself. For instance, I have a few grey hairs. I dye them. I don't let my grey hair show when I'm reading the news.'

In April 2012 the journalist A. A. Gill caused outrage with his comments about the academic and TV presenter Professor Mary Beard. Reviewing BBC2's historical documentary *Meet The Romans* in his Sunday newspaper column he commented that Beard 'really should be kept away from cameras altogether'.

In 2010 he had gone even further in his criticism of Beard: 'For someone who looks this closely at the past, it is strange she hasn't had a closer look at herself before stepping in front of the camera. Beard coos over corpses' teeth without apparently noticing she is wearing them. The hair is a disaster, the outfit an embarrassment. If you are going to invite yourself into the front rooms of the living, then you need to make an effort.' (In 2010 he also called the sports journalist and national treasure Clare Balding 'a dyke on a bike', thus proving that he is not only a misogynist but also a homophobe.)

Professor Beard admitted that she had been hurt by Gill's criticism, but: 'The real point is not what I look like, but what I do. And the response from most viewers to my programmes is that I present interesting, absorbing and enjoyable ones.' Given the paucity of older women on our screens, perhaps we should rejoice that she is there at all.

Gill's attack on Beard was not only offensive but also unprovoked. In the end, everyone seemed to agree that she came out on top – her response, in an article for the *Daily Mail*, was dignified and honest: 'Sure, I don't wear make-up. I have nothing against those who do if it gives them pleasure, but actually I feel happy enough in my own skin not to feel I want to bother with it. I don't dye my hair for the same reason... To the charge of having big, tombstone teeth, I plead guilty. I inherited them from my mum, just as I did her uncompromising double chin. I'm every inch the 57-year-old wife, mum and academic, half-proud of her wrinkles, her crow's feet, even her hunched shoulders from all those misspent years poring over a library desk.'

Miriam O'Reilly, Fiona Bruce, or Beard vs Gill, these are high-profile examples but they matter; this nonsense of women not being allowed to look their age on television is important for all of us.

*

Much of the anxiety surrounding female ageing is linked to keeping one's figure. Not easy, when we're told that our metabolism slows down, we need fewer calories as we age, that we should stay active and supple, despite the hormonal and physical changes of getting older. We mustn't succumb to the middle-age spread – but we shouldn't get scrawny either.

Ironically, given the multiple pressures on women, the best way to look youthful is not to be too thin. So who should we obey: the Ministry of Thin or the Ministry of Fat? As the comedian Miranda Hart says: 'Fat don't crack'. This is an adaptation of the expression 'Black don't crack', meaning that black women tend not to get wrinkles and lines. The supermodel Heidi Klum agrees: 'The ultimate beauty secret for a woman getting older is – don't be too thin! It is always better to have a little meat on your bones. When you are just muscle, you end up being gaunt in the face, and that makes you look older by five or ten years.' (*Self Magazine*, 2012)

She's right, of course: being thin can be ageing. I was criticised for writing, in *An Apple a Day*, that 'anorexia is a young person's game'. I don't take it back because it's true – you can get away with being waif-like when you're twenty-one; when you're fifty-one it looks awful. Physically, female anorexia mimics female ageing in the grimmest way: the thinning hair, crumbling bones and loss of libido; that post-menopausal aridity. All the female hormones dry up (in anorexia and in ageing) and no amount of make-up or surgery can replace the glow of healthy youth.

The journalist Sarah O'Meara recently blogged on the *Huffington Post* website: 'Fat is good for radiant skin. Plump and glowing complexions after the age of 35 tend to belong to one group of women: and they're a size 16. So instead of obsessing about being thin, the best beauty advice would involve large portions of toast and butter.'

Inconvenient but true – anyone on a low-fat diet, i.e. most women at some point in their lives, knows this. Being thin may be good for your figure, and good for designer clothes, but it makes you look ancient. I remember an interview with Courtney Cox, back when she was Monica in *Friends*. She said something along the lines of: with dieting, you have to choose between your body and your face.

In my twenties this was puzzling; now it makes perfect sense. It's like the first time I heard the title of that Nora Ephron book:

I Feel Bad About My Neck – instinctively you understand it. I don't feel bad about my neck – yet – but female ageing does seem to involve a lot of neck-anxiety. My best friend's mother recently had a neck lift in Florida: $5,000 to have her chin, neck and jowls sliced off and sewn up all tight.

The novelist Hilary Mantel tells a lovely story about her mother and our first female Prime Minister: 'My mother, who is the same age as Margaret Thatcher, could never see her in her heyday without remarking, "I wish that woman would go home and look after her neck."'

And the funny-lady on ageing, Nora Ephron, thinks concealment is futile: 'The neck is a dead giveaway. Our faces are lies and our necks are the truth. You have to cut open a redwood tree to see how old it is, but you wouldn't have to do that if it had a neck.'

*

Behind all their personal vanity, women themselves always have an impersonal contempt for woman. (Friedrich Nietzsche)

Clearly, the general age discrimination towards women is unjust. The most logical thing would be for us to unite against sexism, to decide that we're not going to judge other women on their age, appearance, or anything other than merit. Women make up 51 per cent of the global population, so we could be very powerful if we stuck together. However, that's exactly what we don't do. Nietzsche's point holds as true in the twenty-first century as it did in the nineteenth century; too often in ageing, as in the media and the workplace, we are our own worst enemies.

As if critics like A. A. Gill weren't enough, we add our own harsh judgements of other women. Look at the vitriol directed at

Madonna for her relationships with much younger men. Now in her fifties, the pop singer is routinely ridiculed for her love affairs with 'toy boys'; in 2010 she dated Jesus Luz, a man twenty-eight years her junior (incidentally this is the same age gap as that between Rod Stewart and his wife Penny Lancaster, although that doesn't create the same scandal). Madonna is also scorned for working out excessively, for trying to keep her figure and stay youthful-looking, even though that is exactly what we demand of women in the public eye. Most of the scorn is generated by female journalists for female readers.

Even among young women the pressures start early, as in the case of a thirty-two-year-old TV presenter on *The X Factor* called Caroline Flack. In 2011 she committed the sin of having a brief affair with a seventeen-year-old singer from the boyband One Direction. The sin was not in the affair itself, but in the age difference. Questioned about her public vilification Flack later said: 'I think it's 100 per cent harder to be a woman than a man in the public eye. Women should stick together...'

In the case of Madonna, or Demi Moore, or Caroline Flack, women dating younger men provokes moral outrage from the media. *This will all end in tears*, they warn, and it usually does. When it seems to work, as in the case of the artist Sam Taylor-Wood and her much younger husband Aaron Johnson (an age gap of twenty-three years, and they've had children together), the media doesn't know what to make of it. In 2010 Ronnie Wood left his wife for a woman forty-two years younger than him, and the press rolled their eyes indulgently. Boys will be boys...

In the Ministry of Age older women with younger men is strictly *verboten*: this kind of age difference is a red rag to a bull. No matter how glamorous or successful they may be, so-called female 'cougars' are ostracised by society. So when the relationship goes wrong, the older woman seems to deserve the personal misery and public humiliation. How dare they try to be attractive to a younger man; how dare they think their age didn't matter.

*

Nowhere is this sexism-ageism more blatant than on dating websites. One of my closest friends, J, was recently searching for lurve on *The Guardian*'s Soulmates site. You might expect to find a more enlightened class of man on *The Guardian* website: perhaps someone who didn't think a bloke in his fifties should be looking for a pretty little twenty-something; someone who wasn't looking for young totty. You'd be wrong.

We looked at the website and discussed what J should write on her profile. She was hoping to meet someone intelligent, solvent, 'and ideally with his own teeth and hair', but age-wise, she wasn't fussed. In her mid-thirties, she was happy to meet anyone between the ages of thirty and fifty.

As we scrolled through the male profiles, I was shocked at the perfectly open gender-age discrimination. Almost without exception the men specified that they were looking for women a good five to ten years younger than themselves – in some cases, fifteen or twenty years younger. Even more than female body shape, female age seemed to be the determining factor in snaring an eligible man. Up to twenty-nine years old (for women) seemed to be acceptable, but anything over thirty seemed to set off warning bells: *shit, she'll want marriage/babies/commitment.*

This is nothing new: both in research and in real life we know that older men seek younger women – the sugar-daddy, arm-candy phenomenon. The gender-age imbalance is socially accepted, and 'twas ever thus. We're used to seeing rich and powerful men (however unprepossessing) with their beautiful younger partners: think of Bernie Ecclestone, Harvey Weinstein, Donald Trump,

Michael Douglas, Mick Jagger, Hugh Hefner, Bruce Forsyth, Des O'Connor, the list is endless. Of course there are evolutionary reasons for this: younger women tend to be more fertile and therefore more likely to bear your offspring; the biological imperative. But still, as J looked for men who might actually be interested in having a relationship with a woman <gasp> of the same age, the ageism was glaring.

Interestingly, J said that the equivalent of female age is male height – it's the one thing women actually mind about on dating websites: 'I don't mind an odd-looking bloke, even if he's losing his hair, but I filter out all the really short men,' she told me. (A postscript: after a summer of hopeless dates, J met someone amazing, her own age. So there is hope.)

*

So is it all downhill for women? I am trying to think of great things about female ageing, but I find it hard. There are the absences of negatives, I suppose: less insecurity about one's appearance (although many of us feel more insecure, not less); fewer sleepless nights with babies or young children; and some positives: financial security (if you don't experience discrimination at work); a mature and settled marriage (if your husband hasn't run off with a younger woman). There is also the confidence which many older female role models talk about – sexual confidence (ironically as our bodies are starting to sag) and confidence in one's own thoughts and abilities. There is a genuine freedom in not caring what other people think of you. One of the nation's favourite poems is Jenny Joseph's *Warning*, which starts with those wonderful lines: 'When I am an old woman I shall wear purple' – a joyous paean to ageing disgracefully.

*

I had thought that getting older would be harder. The common cultural script tells us that women lose value as they age... Middle-aged women are supposed to mourn the loss of their youthful selves with grief and anguish.

(Naomi Wolf, *The Sunday Times*, 2012)

Long ago I decided that as you grew older, you had to let either your face or your body go. I gave up the body and thereafter spent money on face creams and shoes.

(Fay Weldon, *The Sunday Times*, 2012)

I found myself greatly cheered by Naomi Wolf's robust attitude – armed with her newly revitalised vagina (yes, really) she is clearly dealing with ageing OK. But Fay Weldon's experience seems a little closer to the truth. So how do the rest of us feel about it?

As a child I couldn't wait to grow up. Now, in my thirties, I have started to worry about age. I find myself caring about stupid things like the frown lines on my forehead, and I dread finding my first grey hair. Have I damaged my skin with my teenage sun-worship? Will I regret all those years of not wearing a proper sports bra? Then there are the aches and pains: I've had a painful twinge in my thumb for the last week. A few years ago I would have assumed I'd pulled a muscle; now I'm googling 'osteoarthritis' and imagining my joints seizing up!

And then there's the existential angst – all those things you should have done by the age of thirty – realising you're now too ancient to win any young journalist, scientist or athlete of the year awards. I'm convinced that I haven't achieved enough, that I should have started writing years ago, that other TV presenters are properly trained and

Botox-baby-smooth; that everyone else is more talented and much younger. It's like that anxious niggle as you settle into your pyjamas on a Friday night: is everyone else at some fantastic party?

Quite a few of my friends are older than me, but I do have some female friends in their twenties still. So do they worry about the future? Do they fear the big 3-0, as I fear the big 4-0?

At twenty-seven and 8 days, I don't worry about turning thirty just yet. However, the increasing sun-spots, white hairs and wrinkles do not have me overjoyed. I'm getting better at styling myself as I get older so image isn't really a concern, I think it will depend more on what stage I'm at in my life, e.g. do I have a boyfriend, house, good foundation for a family etc. However if I don't have any of those things then my critique will most likely turn inward and start picking apart everything about myself from the way I look to the way I act and so on. (S)

I'm excited at the prospect of turning thirty. To me, 'thirty' means independent, sophisticated, successful and confident. Whether that will turn out to be true remains to be seen... but I can't wait to find out! The only thing that bothers me with age is how much it seems to affect other people. I couldn't care less how old somebody is, and as clichéd as it is, I think it really only matters how old you feel. A friend told me that the optimum age to start using anti-wrinkle cream is seventeen. I was already twenty-four, so thought it was too late to bother, and have never spent a penny on anti-ageing products. The market is all one big con, and it angers me to see people being taken in by the idea that every aspect of your body has to be perfect and look as young as possible to make you acceptable as a human being. Seriously, what is the purpose of anti-ageing neck cream?! I love people like Maggie Smith and Judi Dench who have embraced their natural looks and still look fabulous, because they are happy and healthy. (D, twenty-six)

As a woman, I feel that my life is mapped out for me in terms of age. Although they're supposed to be empowering, lifestyle magazines put so much emphasis on a woman's thirties that sometimes I feel that your thirties is the only time a woman should be happy with herself. Articles on twenty-somethings I find have a feel of 'oh you must be having so much fun, but don't worry you'll calm down and be happy with yourself one day' and forty-plus is all dressing to disguise your age, how you can still enjoy life, look at these real-life women being happy despite their desperate old age. Apparently your thirties are your sexual/ career/social hey-day – and that's all you get. (A, twenty-three)

Twenty-three years old – imagine being twenty-three again! As George Bernard Shaw said, 'youth is wasted on the young'. If I'm honest, these responses from my twenty-something friends made me feel really... old. And they're sort of meaningless – because what do you know about ageing when you're twenty-three? There is a breezy certainty to extreme youth which recedes with the passing years: we may know more and earn more as we age, but we also learn that life can be a painful, uncertain business. It reminds me of an observation by F. Scott Fitzgerald: 'At eighteen our convictions are hills from which we look; at forty-five they are caves in which we hide.'

To cheer myself up I turned to my friends who are a few rungs ahead on the age ladder. H emails:

Ageing never used to bother me but now that I'm thirty-seven I'm starting to notice tangible signs of old age: extra wrinkles when I smile, creases on my neck that weren't there a few years ago. I'm not worried, exactly, but I can tell I've moved from the 'I'm going to live forever' phase of my twenties into a phase that says 'one day I'm going to be really wrinkly and old'. But then I think that when I'm fifty, I'll think: wasn't I young and flexible and gorgeous when I was forty!

I know what she means. I see photographs from my early twenties and I can't believe how fresh and young I looked. And yet at the time I was probably besieged by all sorts of insecurities. (A reminder that we should appreciate what we have before it's gone.) H continues:

There's a saying: If you're worried about old age, just consider the alternative. I think that's a pretty healthy outlook. And my mum is fitter now at sixty-nine than I am at thirty-seven, so I think there's hope for all of us, even if we can't avoid the wrinkles that are coming our way. Turning thirty was great – it felt like I'd left behind the doubts and fears of my twenties and was ready to emerge into confident womanhood. People are less likely to try to push a thirty-something woman around than a 'girl' in her twenties…

She continues:

I never felt very beautiful as a woman so I haven't noticed a falling-off of attractiveness. I am less confident about baring my skin than I used to be – I feel generally softer and squashier – but I think most of this is, and always has been, in my head, as I see lots of confident women of all ages in shorts and vests. I dye my hair but haven't tried any other anti-ageing treatments. I plan to be honest and go grey one day. But I feel that if I have children, I'll be judged less harshly for being an 'older mother' if I keep my hair looking young – so I won't be giving up the dye any time soon.

Another friend, also thirty-seven, emails about the scarcity of older women in the visual media, in television, film and advertisements:

> *Sometimes I feel angry when I see wrinkly male presenters in their sixties and seventies, and a distinct absence of female presenters of the same age. I think it may very gradually change as audiences continue to get older. I listen to the radio a lot and I feel older women are better represented there, for obvious reasons.* (C)

(Interesting that in the United States, age-phobia has even reached the spoken level. Some US cosmetic surgeons offer the option of a voice-lift: a surgical procedure to make the voice sound younger.) C continues:

> *Another thing that REALLY BUGS ME is films where a young pretty woman falls for a man in his fifties (Richard Gere, Anthony Hopkins, George Clooney) and nobody thinks that's odd. Apart from* The Graduate*, how many films are there where a young man falls for a mature woman?! Meryl Streep should be in loads of rom-coms where hot young men swoon at her feet. She's probably got better things to do, though. Another thing that gets me: TV advertisements for anti-wrinkle cream where the woman using the product is clearly in her early twenties, or is a beautiful older woman (Andie MacDowell, Claudia Schiffer) who's had lots of production magic to ensure there are no lines or wrinkles to be seen. But I just accept these things as being ridiculous, rather than getting overly upset by them.*

J, aged forty-three, tells me:

> *Well... on the one hand ageing doesn't bother me at all as I'm happier in myself than I was at thirty. I'm not affected by media*

images so much as I don't watch TV or read women's magazines – the latter I gave up partly because they are designed to make you feel inadequate and buy more stuff. But I am sad about ageing too – I don't like getting wrinkles or seeing my hair lose its colour. Although I feel fitter than ever, I do feel a little jealous of the beauty of youth sometimes, and of course ageing means there are sad things to come. Age milestones feel big at the time, but then you pass them and forget about them. But I wouldn't say I don't give a toss. Still, I think the confidence you get after forty makes up for lack of youthful looks, and so you don't become less attractive; you're also less needy, I think, in terms of needing to be attractive and perfect-looking – by forty you should know that there are far more important things in life, but you also know enough to enjoy a bit of glamour and flattery from time to time!

*

Age is relative, of course. As a child, grown-ups seem impossibly ancient: you can't imagine being in your forties and still wanting to have fun or still feeling unsure. Adult life seems both boring and predictable – but then you become an adult yourself and find it's nothing like that. There is no age limit to feeling foolish or falling in love; no magic moment when you suddenly become 'grown-up'. Signing your first mortgage documents, or interviewing for an office assistant, even becoming a parent, these don't make you automatically 'grown-up'. That joke about policemen looking so young these days – it's true! The Prime Minister is only five years older than my boyfriend, the Chancellor of the Exchequer was at school with my big brother. Only the other day I realised my dentist was younger than me.

Age isn't fixed, and people really do age at different rates. I'm convinced that having five children has kept my father (now in his eighties) very youthful. Many women in their sixties and seventies are still working out at the gym, and having sex, and sending funny text messages to their sisters: technically they are 'old-age pensioners'. We all have days where we feel fantastic, and other days where we feel as old as the hills.

And then there are other people's reactions. I'm well aware that most men in their twenties don't register me; to them I'm irrelevant, or an old crone. Fortunately I've never gone in for younger men (although I remember the warm glow when one of my little brother's friends called me a 'fit bird'!) Some of the teenage girls who read my column ask my advice 'as an older woman with anorexia' – and that stings. But then female friends in their fifties tell me I'm in my prime, that I've 'barely even started'. One good thing about ageing – there's always someone older than you.

Anyway, who cares? Our society may idolise youth, but youth does not automatically equal beauty. To me, an actress like Kristin Scott Thomas is more stunning than any of the line-free, blank-canvas, younger Hollywood starlets. She has shadows under her eyes and lines around her mouth; her fragile, expressive quality is beautiful. She has experienced life, and it shows on her face.

The actress Susan Sarandon claims that she enjoys the process of getting older, because: 'What you look like becomes less and less an issue and what you are is the point.' I admire Sarandon's self-possession, but I don't share her relish. She may be a confident ambassador for older women, but I think the writer Nora Ephron is more truthful: 'The honest truth is that it's sad to be over sixty.'

*

Of course ageing is not the worst thing that can happen – as my friend H said, 'consider the alternative'. We are lucky to be here at all: healthy and alive. But when you factor in crow's feet, menopausal mood swings, hot flushes and vaginal dryness, age discrimination and invisibility, I don't think it's an easy process for women. But what about men?

It's simplistic to say that men aren't bothered about ageing at all. In the interests of balance, I have tried to canvass male opinion on this matter – but the men in my life have let me down. I talked to my boyfriend about it, then I tried my best male friend, both my brothers, a male cousin and my father. While writing this book I've had no problem engaging these men in conversation about diets, weight, food, female beauty, male bodies – but on the subject of getting older: nothing. Nada. No reaction. Not fussed. Some said they didn't think about their age, except on birthdays, others didn't get it. Did they worry when their friends started getting married and having kids? Nope. Were they anxious about not being 'settled' by the age of forty? Nope. What about the wrinkles and the grey hairs, did they mind them? Nope. 'Who cares' was the most profound response I could elicit.

Telling, isn't it? Men don't fall off a cliff at the age of thirty, or forty, or even fifty. Men can marry later than women – as we've seen from the dating websites, they have a much longer shelf-life – and of course they are not threatened by the ticking time-bomb of fertility. My parents had their fifth child when my dad was in his fifties. Rupert Murdoch became a father again at the age of seventy-two, Rod Stewart at the age of sixty-six – not to mention Saul Bellow at eighty-four and Julio Iglesias Senior at the age of eighty-nine! There are plenty of jokes about male mid-life crises and unsuitable sports cars, but men do not go through a biological menopause. They age, just as women do (and often a lot less gracefully) but they are not stamped with a sell-by date for marriage and babies, as we are.

Nor are societal pressures as intense for men. I'm fortunate in not having those hideous relatives who badger me about when I'm going to get hitched: remember Bridget Jones's Uncle Geoffrey – 'How's your love life Bridget? Can't put it off forever, tick-tock, tick-tock.' Still, any unmarried woman in her thirties is well aware of the expectation: she should at least have a ring on her finger, if not a baby in the cradle. In middle-age a single woman is considered to be on the shelf – she may even be called a spinster – while a single man is still dashingly described as a bachelor.

*

For all the jokes about hot flushes and cougars, and all the fun we have comparing notes with our friends, there is something peculiarly painful about female ageing. As if the menopause weren't physically gruelling enough, a woman's whole identity as a reproductive being is chucked on the scrapheap. A friend told me of the 'hormonal maelstrom' she battles with, the self-esteem issues and mood swings. She comes across as happy and well-adjusted, and yet – 'I only feel normal for a few days in every month,' she says.

Ageing involves a lot of fragility – not just fragile bones – and loss: the loss of physical beauty and sexual power over men, the loss of fertility, the loss of children when they leave home, and often the death of parents. It is a time of vulnerability, and yet you have to be very strong. My mother was right when she told me that getting older is one of the hardest things you face. As Bette Davis said: 'Old age is no place for sissies.'

I am not at this stage yet, but I identify with the feelings of loss. The early signs are there – the inability to drink more than one bottle of Sauvignon Blanc on a school night (hangovers get radically worse with age); the realisation that I can't go to a meeting without putting *something* on my face these days. I now understand why my grandmother loved her 'rouge'. How depressing, to rely on blusher.

Yet it's not all vanity. If I'm honest, my anxiety about ageing is more linked to the knotty issue of fertility: that fear that time is running out. I don't do regret, but I can't help but think of all the mistakes I've made, the years I've wasted and relationships I've messed up. If only I'd sorted myself out sooner, found the right man, got married and had babies in my late twenties, I wouldn't feel so anxious now. *If only*: two of the most pointless words in the English language.

As I explained, wanting a baby was the main motivation for my recovery from anorexia, knowing that unless I gained weight I wouldn't be able to get pregnant. Even so, I'm still quite ambivalent about being a mother: like many women without children, I don't know if I'm ready to surrender my independence just yet. My big sister reminds me that first-time motherhood is a shock – 'but when it happens, you'll deal with it; everyone does. The whole experience is completely overwhelming, but your baby needs you so much that you just get on with it.' She's right, of course.

And we don't all need to have babies. A woman's choice to remain child-free is increasingly acceptable in our society: levels of childlessness rose steadily throughout the twentieth century. According to the Office for National Statistics the proportion of those who are without children has almost doubled since the 1990s. The latest statistics show that a fifth of women in the UK now reach the age of forty-five without having a child, and this figure is expected to continue rising. Among the reasons for childlessness, there are those who have made a conscious 'lifestyle' choice not to have children, those who have delayed starting a family, and those who are infertile.

But time waits for no man (more to the point, no woman) and I can't stay undecided forever. I hear the warning about female fertility 'plummeting' after the age of thirty-five, and it alarms me. When the clock is ticking, it's hard to make rational choices.

*

I know – what a cliché. Another woman in her thirties. The biological clock…

On the one hand I abhor the sexist assumptions made about women in their thirties – don't employ them, all they'll do is get pregnant and demand maternity leave; don't date them, they'll be desperate to get hitched and have babies. I remember my disgust when an ex-boyfriend in his early forties described thirty-something women as 'sperm bandits'. In retrospect, he was rather smug – and after the 'sperm bandit' comment I wonder why I continued with the date, let alone the relationship!

On the other hand, those annoying assumptions are right. Women in their thirties have to get on with it, if they're planning to do it at all. Biology is against us. On her thirty-eighth birthday I asked my friend H about babies and ageing: 'Concerns about fertility? You betcha! But I'm buoyed up by stories of women who have healthy babies well into their forties. And I'm not in despair. Yet.'

*

When she won the first of her two Booker Prizes in 2009, the writer Hilary Mantel was already well into her invisible female years. Reflecting on the shock of being described as 'the fifty-seven-year-old novelist', she wrote in *The Guardian* (August 2009) about the battle-axes of her mother's generation:

'When I was a child, no one supposed that women over 50 were invisible. On the contrary, they blacked out the sky. They stood shoulder-to-shoulder like penalty walls, solid inside corsets that encased them from neck to thigh... They wore vast tweed coats or impermeable raincoats in glass-green, and their legs were wrapped round and round with elastic bandages, so they took up plenty of space in the world; to increase their area they stuck their elbows out...'

Mantel's memories of these 'unyielding, undaunted and savagely unimpressed' women are glorious – a rallying cry for us all to grow fiercer and fatter; to take up *more* space in the world as we age, not less.

I wonder if it's harder to age now than it was for previous generations of women. With the Internet, 24-hour news, and celebrity culture, everything is more visible and scrutinised than before, so the pressure to stay young is greater than ever. Opportunities for women are also more varied – we've never had such financial, social and sexual independence. Survival rates from breast, ovarian and cervical cancer are higher than ever; contraception has freed us from the tyranny of constant pregnancy; and HRT is helping at the other end of the spectrum.

And look at all the instruments we have at our disposal. Make-up is now super-advanced and can do wizard things to our old-lady complexions. With a blast of dry shampoo and a splodge of age-correcting illuminator we can look like we're in control even when we really don't feel it. But the concomitant pressures to 'turn back the clock' with plastic surgery, injections and fillers are also growing. If we could un-invent the cosmetic use of Botox, would we?

As with the Ministry of Thin, and the pressure to be as slim as superwomen with their personal chefs and trainers, so the Ministry of Age exerts pressure to remain as preternaturally youthful as those same superwomen. You know who I mean: Liz Hurley, Cindy Crawford, Kylie, Helena Christensen – and moving up the spectrum, Helen Mirren, Jane Fonda, Sophia Loren. Ranging from their forties to their seventies, these women look far younger than their actual age. Whether it's down to lots of sleep and water, or great genes, or impressive surgery, we'll never really know. But the effect is the same: to make us feel that if these women look young and beautiful well into their menopausal years, why don't we? As Hilary Mantel writes: 'Every media picture of the rare and glowing Joanna Lumley feels like a challenge; why can't you all be like that, why does she look like a princess and you look like a potato?'

Even advances in fertility treatment are a double-edged sword: prolonging our natural reproductive life and producing miracle babies for some women, while simultaneously sweeping others into a world of expensive, invasive IVF, with the risk of repeated failures and unknown consequences.

On the whole, ageing in the twenty-first century is something of a mixed bag. Look at fake nails, fake hair and fake tan: a triumph of beauty science – those gel manicures stay on for months without chipping – but don't they also hamper the feminist cause? How can you do anything with hair extensions down to your knees and glittery talons; how can you expect to be taken seriously when your skin is sprayed the colour of a tangerine?

Nora Ephron (who died in 2012) took an upbeat view of anti-ageing breakthroughs: 'There's a reason why forty, fifty, and sixty don't look the way they used to, and it's not because of feminism, or better living through exercise. It's because of hair dye... Hair dye has changed everything, but it almost never gets the credit. It's the most powerful weapon older women have against the youth culture.'

*

The most powerful weapon? Funny how war-like the terminology of female ageing is: your best defence against wrinkles, fight the fine lines, attack the signs of ageing, shield yourself from this, protect yourself from that. We are painted lady-warriors, sallying forth, armed with our anti-ageing miracle products.

The media, the workplace, even our own fertility, the odds are stacked against women from their thirties onwards. No wonder it feels like a battle. Every year brings more 'maintenance' tasks: more dyeing and plucking, more concealment and concealer. My friend L reduces me to helpless laughter when we discuss getting older; she has this tirade about the whiskers which appeared 'from nowhere' on her chin in her early forties. 'In my thirties they weren't there – then suddenly, boom, they sprouted, fully formed.'

The whiskers are lying in wait... For all but the fortunate few, getting older *is* a fight: against gravity, grey hairs, middle-age spread. We live in a society where ageing involves so much loss: of fertility, influence, sexual power, perceived beauty. So is it really all that negative – are there no redeeming elements to being a woman of a certain age? Back to that article by Naomi Wolf:

'I personally expected that when I entered the middle of my life I would start to mourn my youthful physical self and that... I would feel a sense of existential loss of self when my appearance began to change. But I am coming out with this and hope that many midlife women will join me: those pangs of loss have largely not happened... A great many of us don't feel wistful or rueful about our earlier physical selves. A great many of us really like where we are. I like where I am.'

I was barely a teenager when *The Beauty Myth* came out in 1990, but I have admired Naomi Wolf ever since. My admiration was slightly shaken with the publication of *Vagina* in 2012, but with her forty-nine-year-old pride in her age, with this confident manifesto for maturity, this refusal to panic about ageing, she has won me over once again.

Because really, what's the alternative? If you can't afford regular Botox, the muscles in your face will move (hurrah) and wrinkles will develop. If you can't face surgical intervention, gravity will take its toll on your body. If you don't want silicone implants, breast-feeding your babies will probably leave its mark. If, like me, you don't want to do any of this stuff, if you just want to live your life and not be made to feel 'past it' at thirty-five, forty-five, or even sixty-five, well… we'll just have to age gracefully.

In the words of the well-known aphorism: 'Age is an issue of mind over matter. If you don't mind, it doesn't matter.' Ageing may not be as simple as that – especially for women – but there is no alternative. All we can do is refuse to mind (too much).

*

Ageing, of course, is one of those female Catch-22 situations: we mustn't get old or fat, but being too scrawny is ageing, and anyway who gives a toss – older women are irrelevant. It might be easier to have a cut-off point, a sort of scrapheap threshold, at which all bets are off, the surgery and the hair-dye and the diets can go out of the window, and married, divorced or spinster, we can just get back to living, eating and ageing normally.

If only there was an algorithm which could tell us the exact weight-to-age-to-making-an-effort ratio which the rest of the world would find acceptable. So we'd know when to try to look nice, and when to just disappear into our haggard corner and give up. Maybe some male scientists will invent one.

I'm probably over-thinking all this. And revealing my own superficiality. Of course there are more pressing global issues – but I think ageing is something that women experience quite viscerally. It is one of the most natural, inescapable, and yet painful, things which happens to us. It can involve a profound loss of identity, a leaching away of all that we are: mother, lover, attractive being, and it leaves us with no right of reply. We can at least protest against sexism and age discrimination – however entrenched it is in society and in the workplace, formal legislation does exist – but invisibility is something else. You can't go on a march for being made to feel irrelevant; you can't demand compensation for not being wolf-whistled at (even though you don't want to be wolf-whistled at). You don't believe it when you're young, but getting old is hard – and much, much harder for women.

So what can we do?

A friend of mine who has a seven-year-old son and is approaching her fiftieth birthday has simply lopped a decade off her age! 'It was a school-gate thing – a moment of madness. A couple of mums were talking about their fortieth birthday parties. When someone asked how old I was I just found myself saying thirty-nine instead of forty-nine!'

That's one way to handle it – and why not? When is the last time anyone, except an official, looked at your birth certificate or passport? Even better if we could simply decide not to care about the number. After all, we're living longer: average life expectancy in the UK is 82.6 years for women (and 78.4 for men) so we're barely halfway through our mortal allocation by the time we reach forty. There is plenty more living to be done, whether you feel spritely or ancient in middle age. We might as well do it with confidence.

*

Anyway, who decides what's 'middle-aged'? In a recent discussion on Radio 4's *PM Programme*, two male contributors discussed whether it begins in your forties or fifties these days. The first man, aged forty-three, said he felt 'happily middle-aged'; the second, aged forty-six, said he still classified himself as 'young'.

The only certainty about ageing is that it will happen to us all, unless we die first. I leave the last word to my great-aunt, Virginia Woolf: 'I don't believe in ageing. I believe in forever altering one's aspect to the sun.'

Chapter 10

THE MINISTRY OF MADNESS

I've done a lot of healing, a lot of thinking. I went through a break-up with a man I'd been with for five years and who I planned to marry and start a family with and it was horrendous. I hit rock bottom and went off the rails. I needed to find myself again and I really feel I've done that and turned a corner. I finally feel I'm in a really good place in my life.

(Sarah Harding, Girls Aloud, *Hello* magazine August 2012)

I'm not a *Girls Aloud* fan, but I have a soft spot for Sarah Harding. She has more personality than your average pop princess, and she's clearly had a tough few years. It's easy to dismiss what she says as self-indulgent nonsense, the usual psycho-babble about finding herself, and turning a corner. This is the pop psychology lingo which many celebrities use these days. And of course Harding makes recovery sounds simpler than it is: she swapped her alcohol addiction for yoga, found her inner beauty and learned to love herself again. Life isn't that simple, no matter how rich or famous you are. But it got me thinking about how we describe the toughest times in our lives, and what we actually mean by breakdown.

It's a term we use quite casually, but how do you know when you're having a breakdown? When I think about my own experience of 'mental illness' – another indefinable term – I wonder if I qualify. There was a gradual physical breakdown with anorexia, no doubt, but was there a mental breakdown? How serious does the madness need to get, and is it measured by the individual experience, or the outside world? Probably I'm too inhibited, too 'middle class' to break down properly: I was brought up not to make a fuss. I had plenty of (mostly useless) therapy, but I was never hospitalised. I never seriously attempted to kill myself. Reading *Hello* magazine, I realise that Sarah Harding's experience sounds more exciting: I wonder why I didn't go 'off the rails', why I didn't organise a proper crack-up.

I don't even know what cracking up would entail – not filing my column to *The Times* on time? Not doing my laundry? Taking up smoking again, and drinking too much wine? My friend F told me about her breakdown: 'utterly losing the plot' on the bathroom floor and being carted off to A&E late at night by her girlfriend and mother. It all sounds so dramatic. I think if I rang my parents and said I was having a breakdown, they'd suggest I pop round for a nice cup of tea.

My friend H says:

Speaking personally, I went through a major break-up and felt bloody miserable for some months and then sporadically bloody miserable for a year after that but I still kept working. Having said that, I did turn up to work one day, only to go into my boss's office and say 'I'm just so miserable...' Lovely man, he sent me on a day trip to Wittenham Clumps to cheer myself up, having been through a period of depression himself a year or two earlier. He

THE MINISTRY OF MADNESS

didn't even mark it as sick leave or holiday, just said 'come back tomorrow'. He was just what I needed!

Maybe this is how we deal with someone who is cracking up; maybe it's the best way – a nice cup of tea, a day off walking in the Oxfordshire hills.

No one teaches you what a breakdown looks like; it's not something you learn at school. When do you say 'this is my rock bottom'; how is falling apart measured? Perhaps I wasn't doing enough drink and drugs to go off the rails in style: my breakdown felt more like a slow-motion car crash, over a decade. I think that many people fall apart gradually like this, struggling on day by day, working, semi-functioning, all the while feeling depressed enough to want to die. When there's no sudden crisis, no blood or razors or dramatic overdoses, you can keep going indefinitely, just about holding it together. And that's why suicide is often not a wish to die, but a cry for help – the only way to be taken seriously.

For me, madness was more of a drawn-out whimper than a bang, and that's probably true of most mental illness. Going quietly out of your head and everyone thinking you're just a bit down. Wanting not to be yourself any more. Watching everyone else living the dream. For women this is often linked to one's own body, and despising oneself for the repeated failures to snap out of it, get in shape, lose weight, dress smarter, be someone different. In his novel *Freedom*, Jonathan Franzen puts it beautifully: 'the simplest definition of depression that he knew of: strongly disliking yourself.'

We underestimate how tiring it is, disliking ourselves. We live in our bodies and yet we don't like the skin we're in. *Inside every fat woman there's a thin woman trying to get out* – a joke which rings hollow, when so many of us feel trapped inside the wrong identity. All this disordered eating and body dysmorphia destroys

`

our self-respect. Peace of mind, when you're at war with yourself, is impossible. In the unlikely event that you do, as a woman, feel OK about yourself these days, you're wrong: there is always someone thinner, fitter, younger and more beautiful. Anyway, as the debacle over Samantha Brick (of whom we'll hear more later) reminds us, it's socially unacceptable to be satisfied with yourself.

Female standards of beauty are impossibly high, and male and female expectations are warped by pornography and airbrushing. In this brave new world of cosmetic surgery and anti-ageing treatments, there's really no excuse for getting old and fat. Lift it, dye it, inject it, put it away... Surrounded by images of domestic goddesses, age-defying glamazons and rail-thin models, we always feel we should be doing more, eating less. Taking up less space.

And yet, despising oneself is self-defeating and pointless. No one can turn back the clock. Lie about your age if you want, but we're all going in the same direction. Being constantly hungry is no life at all. Getting thinner doesn't make you happy. The more you starve your body, the more you starve your brain, which in turn makes it even harder to manage your emotions or maintain your self-esteem. In part my anorexia was an apology to the world, for being me, for existing, for feeling all wrong.

*

Remember the Thin Commandments? Taken to extremes, here's where they end up.

1. Never admit you are skinny enough.
2. Binges should only occur a maximum of once every six weeks and must be kept private, if you expect perfection. Purging and excessive exercise MUST follow... otherwise, you're a failure.
3. Never let your stomach growl. You can control it.

4. 10 glasses of water a day, 10 sticks of gum, 10 diet sodas, and 10 cups of black coffee must be consumed on a regular basis for your perfect body's essential needs.

5. Wrist bones are infatuation. Ribs are sexy. Collar bones are beautiful. Hip bones are love. Back bones are submission, but the two bones that connect your ankle to your foot, those are perfection.

6. Flat stomachs are banned; concave stomachs are the only kind acceptable.

7. Fast at least 5-7 days every month, and exercise 7 days a week, at least 2 hours a day.

8. Weigh yourself at least three times a day and hate yourself no matter what the number is.

9. Never give up on what you want most. Ana loves you only if you're thin.

10. Recovery is a sin... but sins are forgiven. Remember obesity is a crime and crimes are on your permanent record FOREVER.

(Source: theanabelles.blogspot.co.uk)

These are the thin laws, and it's this kind of madness which fuels the misunderstanding of anorexia. Most people with eating disorders do not think like this. You may think that doesn't make sense at all, but trust me: the Ana Belles and their 'thin laws' are utterly misguided, and I don't agree with a single one. I may have spent several years living on '10 sticks of gum, 10 diet sodas and 10 cups of black coffee' but I've never referred to anorexia as 'ana'. It's a terrible addiction, not a sister or a friend.

We may not use the terms insane or mad any more, but abnormal, disordered and illness are just as problematic. Yes I was anorexic but I didn't meet many of the strict medical criteria for anorexia. I never thought I looked fat (although many sufferers do experience this) and I never glorified my ribs or collar-bones. People with anorexia are deemed to be mentally ill, but most of them have not lost their grip on reality: they don't actually want to die. There are much easier ways of dying than starving yourself.

I was classified as anorexic because I lost around half my body weight – but the issue of weight loss is another source of misunderstanding and misdiagnosis. In the bible of mental illness, the Diagnostic and Statistical Manual of Mental Disorders (DSM-IV), the criteria for anorexia nervosa is 'weight loss leading to maintenance of body weight less than 85 per cent of that expected'. However, it is possible to experience the mental torment of anorexia even without significant emaciation. You can be a normal weight and struggle with anorexic thoughts. In *An Apple a Day* I mentioned a woman I know who weighs 19 stone, but is still deeply anorexic and fearful of food. Yes, she has regained the weight and more, but she has never recovered in her head.

None of the many people I know with anorexia or bulimia would even look at a pro-anorexia or pro-bulimia website – I never had until today. Those 'thinspiration' sites are dangerous, obsessive and immature. I know my criticism sounds harsh, but I am also full of pity and sadness for these sick individuals. They glamorise anorexia and ignore the breadth and misery of eating disorders. They show slender limbs rather than a woman vomiting food into a lavatory. Of course a waif-like model is a more arresting image than an overweight binge-eater: both conditions are equally destructive but anorexia is seen as more photogenic. But it's not photogenic or glamorous, or at least it doesn't feel that way from the inside.

Here is where language breaks down: the external appearance and the internal experience are worlds apart. I've written an entire book on anorexia and yet I feel I haven't come close to explaining it. Anorexia is complex precisely because it's mental warfare; a constant psychological battle with yourself and your body and your hunger. Any human need for rest or warmth or food must be overcome. Any gesture of kindness towards yourself, any basic care is read as indulgence. Punishment is good – starving oneself yes, but also pain and excessive exercise and loneliness. Anything which isn't painful is weak; anything which isn't punishing is a waste of time. These were the rules which governed me – private rules, inside my head, but just as damaging in their own way as the 'thin laws' on the Internet. Hunger is an addiction as strong as nicotine, alcohol or any drug. Whether it triggers or is triggered by neurological dysfunctions in the brain, we don't yet know, but anorexia involves far more than food restriction. There are powerful psychobiological, physiological and genetic forces at work. Those 'thin laws' are dangerous, not because they will turn anyone anorexic – although there is always that risk – but because they misrepresent this complex condition. They make anorexia sound like a simple desire to be thin. They make it sound like a lifestyle choice.

*

So, if anorexia is disordered eating, what does ordered eating look like? If it's considered mad to starve yourself voluntarily, what is sane? Where is the line between normal dieting and body-hatred, and abnormal mental illness? A reader emailed me recently to ask: 'how quickly did you know you had anorexia?' I answered, truthfully, that I knew from the start. My weight started falling from 9 to 8 to 7 to 6 stone, and I was caught in the trap. But I still don't understand why most women diet and exercise and don't develop anorexia, and I did. There must be a liminal point, a dividing line between sanity and insanity; I'm genuinely perplexed as to where this line might be.

As we've seen, it's normal to be on a diet. A sizeable minority of women value thinness almost more than life itself: a 2011 survey found that nearly one in three women aged from eighteen to sixty-five years would be willing to die younger in exchange for the 'ideal' figure. Up to 16 per cent said that they would swap one year of their life for the perfect body, and 10 per cent would exchange between two and five years (Success Foundation, 2011).

Along with being obsessed with weight loss, it's normal to dislike oneself. You may recall the public vilification of a woman who dared to call herself beautiful. In April 2012 the journalist Samantha Brick wrote an article on the *Daily Mail* website entitled 'There are downsides to looking this pretty: Why women hate me for being beautiful.' Just to give you a flavour of her article:

> *I'm tall, slim, blonde and, so I'm often told, a good-looking woman. I know how lucky I am. But there are downsides to being pretty – the main one being that other women hate me for no other reason than my lovely looks. If you're a woman reading this, I'd hazard that you've already formed your own opinion about me – and it won't be very flattering. For while many doors have been opened (literally) as a result of my looks, just as many have been metaphorically slammed in my face – and usually by my own sex.*

Brick went on to explain that she had been cold-shouldered by friends, jealous wives, and even bosses simply because she was attractive. She concluded, 'women find nothing more annoying than someone else being the most attractive girl in a room'.

Her perceived arrogance caused the article to go viral on social media websites and she became a figure of Internet hatred. The article got 1.5 million hits on the newspaper's website and over 5,000 readers left comments, many of which were offensive, bordering on abusive.

You may have found Samantha Brick's tone smug or self-satisfied. To me, it's not the original article, but the overwhelmingly negative reaction to it, which is most revealing. The vehemence of the comments highlighted just how unacceptable it has become for a woman to feel good about herself or her body; more than that, how outraged people become when we don't hate ourselves.

*

Just as it's become normal to live with constant, low-level self-hatred, so it's normal to be screwed up. I don't know anyone who doesn't have 'issues': a difficult relationship with their mother, a commitment problem, a tendency to drink too much alcohol, or to over-exercise. The rare thing these days is to be balanced or content. So where does all this madness come from?

In part it comes from our over-anxious Western society, a sort of self-consciousness, where any mildly problematic behaviour is classified as a syndrome or a disorder. There is also the fact that we like to have someone or something to blame. In our me-me-me culture, we're used to instant gratification; we expect a pill for every ill. These days, when things go wrong with the trains, or institutions, or a crime is committed, there is usually some form of compensation. *Where there's blame, there's a claim*, right? Similarly when we have personal problems, or act badly, or let others down, we look to the medical community for a reason. And there are more and more reasons being invented every day: the Diagnostic and Statistical Manual of Mental Disorders, contained 112 disorders when it was first published in 1952. It now contains nearly 400 – nearly four times as many recognised mental disorders than sixty years ago. Given that we have higher levels of wealth, health, education and overall living standards than we did halfway through the twentieth century, it seems unlikely that we should be so much madder.

Yes, there is a diagnosis for everything, from night-eating to pathological hoarding to post-relationship embitterment disorder (don't we all know this one?). Someone who spends too much time and money online is labelled a 'compulsive shopper' or an 'Internet addict'; a serially unfaithful husband can blame his 'sex addiction'; a bad relationship can be ascribed to 'partner relational disorder'. Not that these problems do not have their roots in genuine psychological conditions – they may well do – but they're also perfectly normal human behaviours, being greedy, sleeping around, resenting an ex after a break-up. I recently found my boyfriend reading up about 'intermittent explosive disorder' online – a great excuse for his bad temper.

In some ways it's more normal to have 'issues' than not.

I wouldn't dream of suggesting that anorexia is normal, but there is no doubt that disordered eating habits are becoming more widespread. The boundaries between mental health and illness become blurred when it's fashionable to be screwed up. When you look at the range of diets, intolerances and weird food-exclusion regimes out there, you could argue that abnormal eating habits are entirely normal. And among the many non-anorexic women and men I know, the majority could qualify for orthorexia – a preoccupation with healthy food, with exercising a lot, with staying slim. (The label *orthorexia nervosa* literally means 'correct diet' and was coined in 1997 by Dr Steven Bratman to describe an unhealthy fixation with healthy eating.)

But here's the paradox. However mainstream our obsession with weight has become, anorexia goes deeper than this. The women around me may talk about losing weight all the time, but they don't experience genuine distress at eating. They happily eat in public. They find it easier to break their diet than starve themselves. They might feel guilty for eating a chocolate brownie in the afternoon, but the guilt will be fleeting. When I was anorexic I would lie awake and worry about food – I would invent illnesses to avoid any and all eating situations: restaurant meals, Christmas parties, birthday dinners.

So yes, disordered eating is rife, but this is different from an eating disorder. Lots of people are mixed up about food and their bodies, but a diet is still just a diet. Much as I hate to admit it, true anorexia and bulimia nervosa are in a different realm. They're on the other side of madness.

*

So how and why do we cross that line into madness? Is anyone who diets at risk of developing an eating disorder, or is there something else going on?

The causes of anorexia and bulimia remain elusive, but there has been some important neurological research in recent years. It's finally starting to shed light on that dividing line; to understand how eating disorders unfold, why one woman develops anorexia while another does not. At the forefront is the research of Bryan Lask, Emeritus Professor of Child and Adolescent Psychiatry at the University of London, and President of the Eating Disorders Research Society. Professor Lask has come up with a theory he described as like 'lobbing a hand grenade into the discussion' on anorexia. Hand grenade is right...

Using neuro-imagery Professor Lask and his colleagues measured the brain function of young women with anorexia while they were seriously underweight, and then during recovery. Their results clearly indicated that blood flow was abnormal to a structure in the brain called the insula. The insula is like 'a busy train station', because it is connected to most structures in the brain and works as a bridge between the right and left sides of the brain. Because of its complex connections, the insula monitors a wide range of functions including: controlling anxiety, regulating feelings of disgust, communicating feelings of hunger, perceptions of taste, processing the sensation of pain and maintaining an accurate experience of body image. In anorexic patients the insula is not functioning properly: this explains familiar characteristics of anorexia, such as distorted body image and altered perception, as well as the ability to block signals of hunger and pain. It may also explain the rigid thinking – literally, the inability to see the wood for the trees – familiar to anyone with anorexia.

The insula also monitors satiety and bodily awareness. When there's too much of the stress hormone norepinephrine in the insula, as there is in the brains of anorexics, these senses are distorted: some anorexics lose all recognition of what it means to be hungry, some see a fat person when they look in the mirror. Their pain threshold is often elevated. Their fight-or-flight response is permanently switched on. Anorexics exist in a state of near-constant panic, and for reasons no one understands, that panic attaches itself to food.

I interviewed Professor Lask for Channel 4, and found it extremely disturbing, looking at those anorexic brain scans. I could clearly see shrivelled grey matter surrounded by dark areas of cerebrospinal fluid. When the body is starving the brain shrinks quite dramatically, and the fluid fills up the empty spaces. Once again, I remembered struggling through my Oxford Finals, the most punishing academic period of my life, as I felt my mind falling apart. I curse myself for causing all that brain damage. It was both vindicating and frightening to see this on screen.

So why does this matter? We already know that all the major organs shrink in anorexia; no big deal that the brain shrinks too. The big deal is that the insula does not appear to recover. When anorexic patients are restored to a healthy weight, their brain expands back to a normal size, but the problems in the insula remain. This finding shocked Professor Lask and his colleagues. Either the insula is permanently damaged by starvation – which is scary in itself – or the anorexic was born with a dysfunctional insula. It is this finding which may indicate a genetic predisposition to anorexia.

There's no solution yet, but Lask's team recommend that treatment should focus on expanding the insula through Cognitive Remediation Therapy, or CRT. This is less well-known than traditional Cognitive Behavioural Therapy and concentrates on the process of thinking rather than on the content of negative thoughts.

This research is exciting, controversial, but inconclusive. I asked Professor Lask if he realised the significance of his findings to patients, and he assured me that he did. But I didn't mean the scientific significance. I meant the individual significance: what you *do* with the information that you may have an actual neurological dysfunction. On the one hand it's a relief to discover that I didn't imagine it all; on the other hand it's frightening. It could also be disempowering to those struggling to recover. Should they give up on ever being 'normal'?

Whatever the brain dysfunctions detected in those with eating disorders, we may never know which comes first, the anorexia or the madness. Is it a pre-existing condition, or starvation itself which creates the condition? This is impossible to ascertain (without scanning everyone's brains before anyone developed problems). The physical effects of not eating lock you into vicious psychological cycles; lack of food leads to starvation; starvation weakens the body and warps the mind; disturbed thoughts exacerbate disturbed behaviours. Put simply, severe weight loss affects your brain. It makes you unable to think or act rationally or start eating again. And gaining weight does help. When I began to eat, each bite of food made a difference: I felt saner and stronger with every ounce.

*

As previously mentioned, the most authoritative study of self-starvation was carried out by a team of American researchers back in the 1940s. Although it would never have been allowed to proceed today on ethical grounds, the Minnesota Semi-Starvation Experiment (1944–1945) provided a fascinating insight into the physiological effects of starvation. By association, it shed a lot of light on how anorexia develops.

The researchers, led by Ancel Keys, advertised for participants for their study in early 1944. Hundreds of men volunteered to take part, hoping to avoid the wartime draft, and after extensive screening Keys et al. selected thirty-six completely healthy young subjects. None of these men had any kind of unhealthy body image, preoccupation with food or weight, or known mental disorders.

During the first three months of the experiment, the volunteers ate normally while their behaviour, personality and eating patterns were studied in detail. Over the next six months, the men were restricted to approximately half of their former calorie intake. During this semi-starvation phase they lost, on average, 25 per cent of their former weight.

One of the changes immediately observed in the men was a dramatic increase in food preoccupations. They found concentrating on their usual activities increasingly difficult, and became plagued by incessant thoughts of eating. Food became a principal topic of conversation, reading, and even daydreams. As their obsessive food-thoughts increased there was a corresponding decline in interest in sex and all other activities.

As starvation progressed, the number of men who toyed with their meals steadily increased. (You may have noticed this in other anorexics, how they fiddle with food, picking it apart with their fingers, and eating incredibly slowly. This is a common anorexic trait: when you're so hungry and allowing yourself so little food, you want to make it last as long as possible.) Those participants who ate in the common dining room smuggled out bits of food and consumed them on their bunks in a long-drawn-out ritual. Cookbooks, menus, and information leaflets on food production became intensely interesting to men who previously had little or no interest in nutrition or agriculture. In addition to cookbooks and recipes, some of the men began collecting coffee pots, hot plates and other kitchen utensils. One man even began rummaging through rubbish bins.

This general tendency to hoard has been observed in starved anorexic patients and even in rats deprived of food. (I know an anorexic-bulimic woman who has an entire room in her house devoted to boxes of cereal, tins of baked beans, long-life milk. When I asked her what she's saving all this food for, she looks confused: 'I don't know. When I finish it all, then I'm going to start living normally again.' I never got that bad but I sort of understand. She is living as though a world war is about to break out; the hoarding is part of fear, and control, a response to the starvation.)

At mealtimes, the Minnesota Study participants were caught between conflicting desires to swallow their food ravenously and consume it slowly in order to prolong the sensations of taste and smell. Toward the end of starvation some of the men would dawdle for hours over food which previously they would have consumed in a matter of minutes. They would endlessly discuss and plan their day's allotment of food.

During the eighth week of starvation, one volunteer flagrantly broke the dietary rules, eating several 'sundaes and malted milks';

he even stole some penny sweets. He promptly confessed the whole episode in a rush of self-deprecation and humiliation. While working in a grocery store, another man suffered a complete loss of willpower and ate several cookies, a sack of popcorn, and two over-ripe bananas before he could 'regain control' of himself. He immediately suffered a severe emotional upset, with nausea, and upon returning to the laboratory he vomited. He expressed disgust and extreme self-criticism.

Although the subjects were psychologically healthy prior to the experiment, they experienced significant emotional deterioration as a result of semi-starvation. They also showed severe levels of depression and anxiety – some began biting their nails or smoking. Two men developed disturbances of psychotic proportions. One man became so distressed he cut off three fingers of his own hand.

As the six months of semi-starvation progressed, they exhibited many physical changes, including gastrointestinal discomfort; insomnia; dizziness; headaches; hypersensitivity to noise and light; reduced strength; poor motor control; oedema (an excess of fluid causing swelling); hair loss; decreased tolerance for cold temperatures; visual and auditory disturbances, and paresthesias (abnormal tingling or prickling sensations, especially in the hands or feet).

Anyone who has been through anorexia will recognise most of these symptoms.

The men's personalities changed too. Originally quite outgoing and sociable, they became progressively more withdrawn and isolated. Humour and the sense of comradeship diminished amidst growing feelings of inadequacy. The volunteers' contacts with women also declined sharply during semi-starvation. Those who continued to see women socially found that the relationships became strained. 'It's almost too much trouble to see her even when she visits me in the lab,' one man said. 'It requires effort to hold her hand. If we see a show, the most interesting part of it is contained in scenes where people are eating.' Pursuing any kind of romantic or sexual relationship with women simply became too much effort.

After the six-month semi-starvation period the men were placed on a re-feeding programme, but the research notes show that the problems continued: *Subject #20 stuffs himself until he is bursting at the seams, to the point of being nearly sick and still feels hungry; #120 reported that he had to discipline himself to keep from eating so much as to become ill; subject #1 ate until he was uncomfortably full; and subject #30 had so little control over the mechanics of 'piling it in' that he simply had to stay away from food because he could not find a point of satiation even when he was 'full to the gills.'... 'I ate practically all weekend,' reported subject #26. 'I would just as soon have eaten six meals instead of three.'*

Clearly, extreme psychological changes had taken place in these men. Even while they were gradually being restored to a healthy weight, they were unable to recover from their obsession with food. Their bodies never got over that period of starvation. Their minds became permanently hardwired to think it was never enough, there was never enough food, they had to eat, eat, eat or they would starve to death.

The single most astounding finding of this study was that many of the symptoms once thought to be primary features of anorexia nervosa are simply symptoms of starvation itself.

It's crucial to remember: these were psychologically and physically healthy young men. They were normal. However unethical the Minnesota experiment was – it would not be authorised today – it shows that anorexia and bulimia are psychological diseases with clear physiological causes. Our bodies are evolutionarily wired for survival, and by consciously starving we create the conditions for eating disorders to take hold.

I find Minnesota interesting but perplexing too. It seems both to contradict and to support the neurological and genetic anorexia research of recent years. Cycles of abnormal thoughts and behaviours in the Minnesota men (who felt no previous cultural or personal pressure to be thin) were triggered by semi-starvation. On the face of it, it seems that simple: under extreme dietary restrictions these young men were acting just like anorexic young women.

Which bring us back to the question of heredity and madness; cultural pressures and thin idealisation; personal mistakes and lifestyle choices and diets gone wrong. Which comes first, the eating disorder or the starvation? From my own experience of anorexia, I honestly can't say. Professor Lask's research suggests that anorexic brains are not functioning like normal brains; Minnesota seems to suggest that starvation is the trigger which fires the anorexia gun.

*

And the reason all this matters? Because if women desire above all else to be thin, we need to understand what food restriction can do to our brains. Many women will be fine, just dieting. Others will develop severe eating disorders. We need to understand the triggers, traumas and possible long-term consequences, because they may last a lifetime. The behaviour of those previously healthy young men sounded pretty mad, right? When you develop anorexia or bulimia nervosa, you cross from the normal, healthy world into this realm of madness. It is so hard to cross back.

Chapter 11

THE MINISTRY OF SUCCESS

Most of us won't come into contact with the Ministry of Success on a day-to-day basis. This department doesn't concern itself directly with the average woman, only with the crème de la crème – the actresses, models, athletes, singers, TV presenters and other celebrities, wives and girlfriends of famous men, minor royals – the richest and glossiest of womankind. But just because most of us will never attain those lofty heights doesn't mean we aren't affected by them. On the contrary: these lovely creatures are hugely influential. This is where the trickle-down effect comes into play: the comparisons, the dissatisfaction, the sense of inadequacy. Never mind their teams of beauticians and nannies, personal trainers and chefs. If they can be that perfect, why can't we?

It's more than half a century since Wallis Simpson uttered those chilling words: 'A woman can never be too rich or too thin.' In the Ministry of Success, it's never been truer. Modern women in the public eye, almost without exception, slim down as their success increases, and it seems to be a peculiarly female trend.

Look at three of the most high-profile women in the UK today: Samantha Cameron, wife of the Prime Minister; Kate Middleton, aka Princess Catherine, Duchess of Cambridge, wife of William our future King; Victoria Beckham, former Spice Girl, fashion designer, wife of footballing superstar and national treasure David Beckham. A graph of their weight and shape would show their slimness in inverse proportion to their influence: as their fame has increased, their weight has decreased.

Logically this doesn't make sense. Everything we associate with success is about growth. Consider the linguistics of power: burgeoning celebrity, greater fame, growing riches, mounting popularity, higher profile, growth in stature, bigger fan-base, global expansion and influence. So why the female law of diminishing returns; why as women grow they must shrink?

Much of it comes down to control. The more slender your body, the more evident your self-control. Being hardcore in your workouts and disciplined in your diet demonstrates your inner steel like nothing else. If you're visibly 'struggling with your weight' you are all too obviously not on top of things. If you can't control your appetite and your body, how can you control the rest of your life? Flabby doesn't radiate success, it's that simple.

And the figures back this up: slimmer women all over the world are paid more highly, and climb the career ladder more quickly, than their larger counterparts. Countless studies indicate that men generally rate slimmer women as more sexually attractive. This may be because in evolutionary terms we are programmed to associate people who are overweight with an increased risk of health problems. Or it may be because slimness is increasingly rare, and therefore genetically more desirable. Economists and sociologists also recognise this 'beauty premium', whereby thinner women, who are perceived as more attractive, are promoted more quickly in all professions. US researchers have dubbed this the 'plainness penalty', which punishes below-average looks with earnings of 9 per cent less an hour.

Nor is this just the case in the fashion and beauty industries, where appearance could be seen as relevant: for women, being perceived as attractive is of overwhelming importance in every walk of life. And it's not just at work: research has shown that attractive children are more popular and perform better at school, and attractive people are found guilty less often in court.

Interestingly, men's career prospects improve as they *gain* weight: unlike women, thinner men tend to earn less than male workers of average weight. Proof that we don't equate extreme slimness with attractiveness in men.

So, sexism, size-ism, body fascism? Whatever. For all we may rage against the machine, it seems that we don't follow through. When women come into the public eye, almost without exception they begin to lose weight. Think of the former model Sophie Dahl, the food writer Nigella Lawson, the singer Adele (who was described by Chanel boss Karl Lagerfeld as a pretty girl but 'too fat'). The pressure to conform is immense. Of course these women have the right to slim down for health or any other personal reasons. But it leaves us with this conundrum, that of the larger role model who 'embraces her curves', swears she is comfortable in her body, loves her food, that she won't be bullied into losing weight, and then... does precisely that.

Our messages are mixed: on the one hand we want them to be larger, like so-called 'normal women', and yet we bang on endlessly about their size. As the media obsessively monitors the body shape of female celebrities – their incredible curves or their shrinking frame, their gym visits or fast-food habits – we seem no closer to understanding how we feel about weight and women and our waistlines.

*

From comedians to newsreaders to politicians, women's bodies are under surveillance. It's not just models or actresses these days – any woman in the limelight is fair game. The constant scrutiny must be hard to handle. I had a taster of this kind of body-bashing after a *Newsnight* appearance on BBC2 in 2012. Bear in mind that I'd done very little television at this point; that I was fairly anxious about saying something coherent in a complex debate about NHS funding for eating disorder treatments; that I was debating with the Rt Hon Stephen Dorrell MP, Chair of the Health Select Committee. And you know, *Newsnight* and Kirsty Wark and half a million viewers!

I'm aware that in speaking out about anorexia my appearance will be scrutinised even more closely than the average woman. Anorexia is a highly visible condition – despite the fact that it's a mental illness, there are expectations about what it looks like. So maybe I shouldn't have been surprised, the day after *Newsnight*, to see comments on Twitter including: 'Call that anorexic? She didn't look that thin to me', and another: 'Urgh, u still way too skinny. Lollipop head, matchstick arms, FFS eat something girl.' Quite apart from the irrelevance of these comments to the NHS debate, it showed how tricky it is to be in the public eye.

That was my first exposure, but I've since appeared as a co-presenter on the Channel 4 series *Supersize vs Superskinny*. If ever there was an experience to toughen me up, that was it! Every programme I'd see tweets about my appearance – specifically my weight – and at first they upset me deeply. The week I interviewed young men about the rise of male eating disorders, I read on Facebook: 'She still seems very gaunt.' Written by a man!

I used to try to understand: what would impel someone to post their negative opinions online? Don't they consider other people's feelings? Don't they feel mean? But it's not rational – and the hyper-visual, super-connected world of the Internet doesn't help. We see hundreds of images of women every day, and anyone can air their views simply by clicking on comment or post. As soon as I decided that I wouldn't dwell on nasty tweets, or try in any way to reason with them, it became easier. Now I have a rule: read once only, delete if possible, and never respond. If it's particularly unpleasant I will block the tweeter, otherwise I try to forget it.

And yet it's hard not to take it to heart: most of us civilians are not used to having our appearance scrutinised in the court of public opinion. Of course it feels incredibly personal, but it's not really – just thoughtless anonymous twittering, born out of jealousy or boredom. And all women are targets. Anorexic or not, any public exposure leads to the same old criticism, that you're too thin, or not thin enough.

But why do women lose weight as their stature grows, while men do not? Whatever their profession, age or appearance, there is something about being in the public eye which gets to them all in the same way, eventually. My instinctive answer to this is: it's anxiety. I say instinctive because I've been there: I know the gnawing, racing, jittery feeling which not only stops you from eating much, but also ramps your adrenalin up to dangerous levels. For me, it was a self-perpetuating loop of anorexia and starvation, constant exercise, then addiction to the hungry highs and exercise endorphins. The less I ate, the harder I pushed myself; the thinner I got, the more unable I was to get off the manic treadmill.

This is why I watched the run-up to the Royal Wedding in 2011 (of Prince William and Kate Middleton) with alarm: specifically those intrusive paparazzi shots of the 'shrinking' Kate. Like many others I felt uncomfortable at the gleeful/concerned reports of anorexia – but I don't agree with them. I don't think you develop anorexia like that, overnight. Even though our situations are completely different, I could understand why the weight was 'falling off' Kate Middleton – sheer pressure and anxiety and nerves. Just as women tend to gain weight as they settle into long-term relationships because they feel cosy and relaxed, so the constant glare of the media spotlight must make you hyper-vigilant and constantly on edge. For someone as high-profile as the Duchess of Cambridge there are few opportunities for curling up on the sofa in her PJs, eating takeaway pizza.

Getting ultra-thin is also a defence mechanism against the flashbulbs. Female celebrities are extremely vulnerable in the full media glare – you catch this wariness in their eyes, the protective clutching of handbags or babies to their frail bodies, the way Victoria Beckham never smiles. For all the aspects of their lifestyles we might envy, their wealth, success or beauty, fame is a disorienting bubble to inhabit. Being thin allows them a measure of control – and when you're in the public eye, there isn't much else you *can* control. They may be ridiculed for their latest outfit or hairstyle but at least no one can call them fat.

Rightly or not, fat women are seen as approachable, jolly, insulated; thin women as hard, unyielding, self-sufficient. Being very lean, paradoxically, acts like a suit of armour: I have experienced this. When I was skeletal I never hugged anyone, afraid to let the outside world in, constantly vigilant about letting my guard down. In contrast, fatter women are seen as good huggers: mums, best friends, providers of chocolate brownies and love.

A reader recently emailed me a mantra from a blog which glorifies weight-loss. It simply says: 'So that in pictures, any angle is a flattering angle.' For a woman, this needs no explanation.

*

So slimness equals success: you're training hard five times a week, eating only organic food, body-brushing every morning, and losing weight: does that mean you've made it? Sadly not. Because really successful women have a lot more than this. It's no longer enough just to have the perfect body. You also need the perfect life. And that means not only the fabulous career, close female friends and family, but also the idyllic home life.

Husbands and babies are making a comeback in the twenty-first century. After the free love of the 1960s, the bra-burning of the 1970s, the working girls in power suits of the 1980s and the hedonistic 1990s, marriage began to look staid and boring. Proper celebrity meant dating rock stars and snorting cocaine and messy divorces.

But now, in the twenty-first century, marriage and home-making is back in fashion. Look at Lily Allen, settling down and moving to the country and having babies. Taking her husband's surname! At the peak of her success she decided, in her mid-twenties, to step back from the whole 'rude-girl' thing. She announced she was giving up singing, and repeatedly told journalists that all she wanted was to get married and bake cakes and start a family.

These days it's more enviable to boast about your strong, stable relationship than your wild nights out. Being happily married is the new rock and roll. Look at Kate Middleton: well-groomed, well-behaved, always smiling, a template for the perfect 'surrendered' wife. Since their wedding, Prince William has continued his career in the RAF. Kate has no career except that of being the Duchess of Cambridge, wife of the future king, and mother of a royal baby. Every aspect of her life is scrutinised by the world's media, and she lives surrounded by Royalty Protection Branch officers.

At the Wimbledon finals in 2012, comparisons were drawn between Kate Middleton and Kim Sears. Like Kate, Kim is the long-term partner of a famous man, the tennis player Andy Murray. Like Kate, Kim is glossy of mane, immaculately dressed, always discreet and appropriate. They both wear sensible outfits from Hobbs or Jigsaw or Reiss, with tan tights and not-too-high nude heels. Kim Sears actually has her own business painting portraits of pets, but that is not what she is known for. Kim and Kate must follow their menfolk around the world, and they must never express their own opinions or step out of line. No matter how many tennis matches or charity functions they attend, they are never seen tipsy or tired or wearing too short a skirt.

Their decorum is entirely appropriate for their public roles. But it's an interesting phenomenon, this fame-by-proxy. While Kate, at least, made the decision to marry into the royal family, Kim Sears chose no such public role. Why should she be so relentlessly photographed: shouldn't the tennis match, or at least Andy Murray, be the real story? The media have fallen in love with the way these women look, but we know almost nothing about their real personalities. What does it mean to have your appearance, your body, weight and shape so intensively analysed? Who knows how it makes them feel?

Whether Kate actually wanted a career, or whether she finds her royal duties fulfilling in their own right, we can never know. What is clear is that she lives at the epicentre of a media storm. A change of hairstyle – is her fringe a few inches shorter? – a recycled outfit – did she wear that coat-dress three years ago? – makes national headlines.

In their usual mixed messages, the media portray Kate both as 'having it all' – the man, the money and the status – while at the same time objectifying her as mere tabloid fodder. And it's not only the tabloids: respected broadcasters like the BBC focused on her 'bump' when she appeared in public in the early stages of her pregnancy, their cameras actually zooming in on her stomach when she was visiting a woman's refuge. The fact is that Kate never chose to be a role model – it is the media who have elected her as their new ambassador of feminine perfection.

It will be interesting to see what the next generation of women aspire to, in terms of life, relationship and career choices. Feminists have detected a worrying subservience in modern young women and the role models they admire. Cherie Blair, wife of former Prime Minister Tony Blair, and a successful barrister in her own right, spoke about this at a Fortune's Most Powerful Women conference in 2012. She criticised young women who give up personal ambition and self-sufficiency to marry rich men, warning them that this was no way to find fulfilment. Many women, now in their sixties and seventies, who have participated in the battles of feminism in their own lifetime have echoed these thoughts.

Is this a new kind of female obedience? Are these young wives and girlfriends the modern version of the 1950s housewife? It's impossible to know what goes on in private relationships – and unfair to single out Kate Middleton or Kim Sears. However, the set-up is symptomatic of a growing breed of modern women: confident and educated in their own right, but happy to be an accessory. They believe that having a rich husband, a beautiful house and perfect body is enough.

Louise Mensch, the ultimate successful woman, a bestselling novelist, Conservative MP, mother of three, and self-proclaimed feminist, recently gave up her political career and moved her children to New York where her second husband is based. Was this a betrayal of the feminist cause; was Mensch sacrificing her own ambitions in order to be a good wife and mother? To me, the decision to move to New York, to be with the man she loves, to write her books, sounds pretty liberating...

*

It's hard to draw any conclusions, because not all women in the public eye have stopped achieving in their own right. For every well-behaved young wife there's a wild Rihanna making millions from her music; for every trophy girlfriend there's an inspirational Jessica Ennis winning Olympic Gold, or Zadie Smith writing books, or Jo Swinson being elected to parliament at the age of twenty-five. Clearly the distinction between surrendered wife or feisty feminist is overly simplistic: these are shorthand media terms, and they fail to recognise the many shades in-between. Journalists love to polarise the debate, pitting so-called career girls against stay-at-home mums. The distinction isn't that black and white: society is full of successful women, both civilian and celebrity, who combine work with motherhood. Anyway, why should it be one or the other? It isn't for men.

Perhaps we shouldn't give up on women just yet – many are playing the long game. When you look at the achievements of previous wives of famous men, there is cause for optimism. Hillary Clinton, for example, was the First Lady of the United States from 1993 to 2001. Despite being a top lawyer in her own right, she was very much in her husband's shadow. But as Bill Clinton has stepped back from public life, Hillary's star is in the ascendancy: she was a high-profile senator, and then served as Secretary of State from 2009 to 2013. She was a leading candidate in the 2008 Democratic presidential nomination and, though unsuccessful, is seen as a likely future US president.

Or look at Sarah Brown: wife of the former prime minister Gordon Brown. Having stepped back from her public relations career in order to concentrate on her husband's political ambitions, since he left office her profile has risen. She has published a book, runs various charities and was recently elected as a non-executive director for the luxury department store Harrods. Even Victoria Beckham, for so long decried as the ultimate footballing WAG, is now a highly successful fashion designer and mother of four who has worked incredibly hard for her success. In ten years, Michele Obama may well be involved in a new career while her husband will be the ex-president. Look at the women you know in your own life, think of the newsreaders, actresses, politicians and businesswomen who have children and work, or who are older and inspirational. It's clear that female success can come later on, or in a different way.

Despite all this, the situation in the mainstream media is pretty depressing. We see a lot of emphasis on appearance over intellect and ambition. On television, in films and magazines, women are still defined in terms of their relationships, who they're dating, engaged or married to. Maybe female ambition is a casualty of the recession – maybe we're worn out with working, and fed up of hearing that women can have-it-all; maybe feminism feels futile, and we're tired of striving. Successful, beautiful women get the man and the ring on their finger. Domestic bliss is back in fashion.

*

Once the nuptials are over, successful women start having babies. And this is where the Ministry of Thin rears its head again. The modern woman, who has worked so hard to achieve the perfect body, and marry the perfect man, must now conduct the perfect pregnancy. If you're famous, the paparazzi will be focused on your bump at all times (as demonstrated by the treatment of the Duchess of Cambridge). If you're a civilian, every woman's magazine you read will be full of pictures of other pregnant women. Whatever your status you'll be aware of how the golden pregnancy *should* look: a small bump, neat and round, glowing skin and hair. You should probably fit into your skinny jeans until at least seven months, and certainly no swollen ankles, hormonal break-outs or billowing maternity wear. Platform heels until the final trimester.

I'm exaggerating, but you know the sort of thing. Claudia Schiffer, supermodel and mum-extraordinaire, 'confessing' that she lost weight during her pregnancies. Actresses whose stomachs barely show until five or six months along. Celebrities snapped on the beach in bikinis, with their gorgeous husbands kissing their photogenic bump, not a stretch-mark in sight.

Pregnancy used to be the stage in a woman's life where she could forget about her figure. Pregnant women would console each other over the biscuit barrel – 'after all, we're eating for two'. The media is full of scare-stories about what you should and shouldn't be eating and drinking and doing. My mother, who had her five children during the 1970s and 1980s, often advised my big sister to be less anxious about what she ate during her first pregnancy. Thinking back to previous generations, let alone the whole of human history before them, expectant mothers worked, smoked, drank copious amounts of alcohol and coffee, and ate unpasteurised cheeses and cured meats. They weren't afraid because they didn't know of the risks (and their babies were born perfectly healthy).

The Internet is a mecca for pregnancy paranoia. One of the top pregnancy Google searches is: 'Is it safe to dye your hair while pregnant?' The Babycentre website recommends that a normal healthy woman needs 'no increase in calories in the first and second trimesters', and only around 200 calories in the third trimester. This is a surprisingly small amount – barely an extra slice of toast! The weight issue looms large for pregnant women, and modern midwives seem to be obsessed with policing the extra pounds. I've had female friends who have been warned they are gaining too much, and others who have been told they're not gaining enough and the foetus is too small. When you're ravenous the whole time and eating more than usual, or nauseous with morning sickness and throwing up, weight control during pregnancy can't be easy.

For fun, I just tried out the 'pregnancy weight gain estimator' at the Babycentre website – give it a go! I entered my height and weight and here is what it said: 'You will probably gain 12.7 kg – 18.1 kg during your pregnancy. If you gained the average of this range, this is where the weight would go: uterus 1.3 kg, breasts 0.5 kg, blood 1.7 kg, water 2.2 kg, fat 4.4 kg, foetus 3.4 kg, placenta 0.9 kg, amniotic fluid 1.1 kg.' The perfect measurements for the perfect pregnancy.

*

There is a worrying phenomenon known as 'pregorexia'. As the name suggests, this is anorexia and extreme anxiety over body weight during pregnancy and early motherhood. Pregorexia is one of the latest crop of invented 'exias' (like tanorexia or drunkorexia) – a flippant term for a very real condition. Here's how a 'pregorexic' blogger described her experience: 'For me, pregnancy was a nine-month battle in which I lived in a dissociated state from my body, horrified by my expanding self that protested every ounce of weight I gained. I did not experience the freedom to eat for two; rather, I experienced the restriction of starving for two.'

On *Supersize vs Superskinny* I interviewed a young mother who developed an eating disorder during her first pregnancy. By the time she was nine months pregnant, she was so underweight that she and the baby nearly died because she was too weak to push her out during labour. She now has two young children and is still in and out of an eating disorders unit, struggling to maintain a healthy weight.

Clearly, anorexia in pregnancy is serious: it can result in low birthweight, premature birth or even miscarriage. However, having an eating disorder does not make you a bad mother, and it doesn't necessarily harm your baby. I know many anorexic women who have had babies while restricting their diet and exercising more than might be advisable. I also know a woman with severe bulimia who binged and purged throughout three pregnancies and has three robust little boys. I'm in no way condoning this – I hate to think of anyone making themselves sick, least of all while they're pregnant – but the female body is very resilient. However much we would wish otherwise, bulimia and anorexia can and do continue during pregnancy. Generally, the baby will take what it needs from stores of nutrients in the mother's body as well as from her daily diet. In situations of drought, famine, war and poverty, women continue to conceive and give birth to healthy babies. The female body is miraculously designed to protect its unborn child (although of course if a mother's nutrient stores are low, this can lead to deficiencies in calcium, vitamin D and other essential nutrients).

There is an assumption that anorexia and motherhood are mutually exclusive, that anorexics, freakishly thin and often infertile, do not get broody. I understand this: extreme thinness does not 'look' maternal or nurturing or soft. Anorexics do not have child-bearing hips or welcoming bosoms, the physical attributes we associate with love and motherhood. Mixed up with the misconceptions are the physical facts, from amenorrhoea to low oestrogen levels to thin uterus lining (which makes it difficult for an embryo to implant). Put simply, the womb stops preparing itself as a cosy place for the embryo. When you're eating barely enough to sustain yourself, the body can't risk creating a new life. But you can be skinny and maternal.

A few facts. The chances of getting pregnant *after* anorexia are good. Impaired fertility is one of many health complications of anorexia, but long-term sufferers, even those who have not menstruated in years, usually go on to recover their fertility once normal weight has been achieved. Having an eating disorder doesn't guarantee you'll have problems in pregnancy.

*

Like many women, I find the idea of pregnancy both scary and thrilling. On the one side, unavoidable weight gain, body changes, increased appetite, food cravings, loss of control; on the other side, the amazing experience of motherhood.

But just as every pregnancy is different, so every anorexic's experience is different. Some women find that being pregnant exacerbates their anxiety; others find it curiously therapeutic. I asked some female friends with eating disorders how they coped while they were pregnant.

L, now fifty-six, suffered from anorexia throughout her twenties, and went on to have two healthy children:

> *For me the pre-pregnant bit, once I first got my periods back, was much harder than the pregnancy. The uncertainty of it all and the combination of newly active hormones is a tricky cocktail. Your body is getting ready for the biggest event of its life and your emotions are expected to keep up... I remember almost gritting my teeth as I tried to maintain my food intake.*

Once she conceived, L found eating less of a struggle, because she felt validated to feed herself properly:

> *When I became pregnant, the thought of my baby diminished my fear of weight gain. I couldn't wait for the bump to appear – my husband used to laugh when I insisted on standing sideways in photos! I never viewed my bump as a threat.*

L's pregnancy was the spur to put anorexia behind her for good, but it's not always the case. J, now thirty-nine, gained enough weight to conceive, but admits that she struggled with disordered eating through three pregnancies:

> *I know it's terrible but I was vigilant about my diet – I wanted a small, neat bump, I couldn't cope with the idea of getting fat all over. I ended up putting on around two stone with each baby, and they were fairly light at birth, but I made sure I ate the right nutrients, and took every prenatal supplement going! My little boys are taller than average so I don't think I harmed them, but I sometimes feel guilty even now. Pregnancy just seemed a dangerous time, like I'd balloon if I wasn't careful.*

And what do the experts think? I ask my former psychiatrist, and as usual he doesn't pull his punches: 'It's not a good idea for a non-recovered anorexic patient to become pregnant.' Among the reasons, he cites the 'high rate of foetal malnutrition with raised foetal death rate, and significant difficulties with weaning. The answer is to recover from the eating disorder, especially in terms of weight and eating, then try for a baby and get support with accepting body-shape changes during pregnancy – and after the birth, when the feeding issues may occur. Don't allow doctors to give you hormones or IVF because that may just be avoiding the difficult issue of anorexic recovery before conception.'

Sadly, you *can* maintain anorexia through pregnancy. While it may not necessarily harm your baby's health, it may affect their relationship with food. Just as we now understand the importance on the baby of maternal nutrition long before conception, so it seems that unresolved psychological disturbances may reverberate long after birth. Observational studies of anorexic women and their babies (like Hilda Bruch's 1973 *Eating Disorders: Obesity,*

Anorexia Nervosa, and the Person Within) refer to 'conflictual mealtimes', with mothers 'unable to distinguish somatic, bodily sensations such as hunger from emotional feelings such as affection and anger.' Put simply, these women are extra-tense around food. But there is still relatively little known about the long-term consequences of anorexia in pregnancy.

So what's the answer? Is it enough to be aware of the risks, to optimise your nutrition, to seek support during and after pregnancy – or does anorexia make you unfit for motherhood? I love babies: even when I weighed five and a half stone I never doubted that I'd be a mother one day. For me, the desire for children has been the greatest motivation in my recovery.

Through my *Times* column I've received advice from many women, but the one that sticks in my mind is this: 'Please make sure that you're truly better before embarking on motherhood. You need so much strength, mentally and physically, to cope with having a baby.' The stranger's words hinted at something to do with emotional recovery, resilience, maturity, something which goes much deeper than just eating more.

The roots of anorexia run horribly deep. During recovery, I sort of dismissed those who told me to slow down and recover first. The anorexic mindset is ambitious, perfectionist, impatient: once I decided to beat anorexia I wanted immediate results: blooming health, neat pregnancy, adorable newborn. Talking to other anorexics it's clear that motherhood isn't just about those nine months, the weight gain and the bump. It's not even about eating for two. Being ready to be a mother – with all the chaos, physical changes and yes, food, it entails – is quite different from being fertile or getting pregnant. It's recovery – true, psychological recovery – which matters to an unborn baby, not just conception.

An old friend suffered with severe anorexia for fifty years, and has finally overcome it at the age of seventy-four. I once asked her whether it was worth it, being thin all those years but missing out on having a family. Her reply brought me to tears: 'Too late for periods, too late for babies, I am grateful I can enjoy food again. But I still feel a great sadness when I think about the children – and grandchildren – I might have had, if only…'

*

Anorexia and bulimia are extreme cases, of course – I'm not confusing the body-anxiety many healthy women experience in pregnancy with these serious conditions. But in the Internet age, pregnancy is simply more visible. In an endless, rolling stream of paparazzi shots, we're privy to every stage of the perfect celebrity pregnancy, then the perfect post-partum bounce-back. And this pressure to shed the 'baby weight' straight after birth is making a lot of new mothers very miserable.

The other day, a female colleague at work said: 'That Bollywood actress, she had her baby what, a year ago? She's taking her time shifting that weight.' It wasn't intended maliciously, but it made me think. None of us knew whether the baby was a girl or boy, and it didn't much matter; the point was whether the actress was back in shape. In the modern media, pregnancy and recovery is the main event, like some weird form of performance art. Successful modern women have perfect marriages and babies, yes, but the baby can seem like a sideshow, an irrelevance.

So how did pregnancy become such a thing? Where did 'yummy mummies' spring from, and how did men start referring to MILFs (Mothers I'd Like to F***) and even GILFs? How did motherhood get hot?

Arguably one could blame Demi Moore. She kick-started this whole stunningly-pregnant thing with her naked cover shoot for *Vanity Fair* back in 1991. Called the 'mother of all magazine covers', even concealed in a brown paper bag by some magazine stores in the US, it led to a series of copycat covers (including pregnant Britney Spears and Christina Aguilera).

'It did seem to give a little bit more permission to feel sexy, attractive when you're pregnant,' Demi Moore said at the time. 'But I really didn't expect for the response to be what it was. I was pretty shocked.' As with Victoria Beckham, Demi has been vilified by the media – she's too thin; she's spent over a million dollars on cosmetic surgery; she's mutton dressed as lamb; she's getting old (how dare she). Demi was roundly condemned for marrying Ashton Kutcher, fifteen years her junior, then publicly ridiculed when the marriage finally failed. It angers me that this should be so. Of course there are biological and social factors here, but younger women marry men fifteen or twenty years their senior all the time, with no comment or moral censure. Ashton Kutcher's infidelity and their eventual divorce may well have been inevitable, but that doesn't make the situation funny, or Demi Moore's heartbreak any less real. She may be a rich Hollywood actress, but she's still a woman – and ageing is hard. When she became skeletally thin during their break-up, when she was allegedly admitted to rehab with anorexia, when she was reportedly 'calling him up to twenty times a day' while he was on holiday with his new twenty-something girlfriend... I felt very sympathetic.

Nonetheless, that *Vanity Fair* cover made pregnancy a whole lot more challenging for women. If you haven't seen it (google it) it's a tender, maternal image. She's cradling her seven-month bump and she looks beautiful. Not hormonal or grouchy or swollen. And undeniably sexy.

Not all women feel sexy when pregnant, but somehow it's become part of a successful pregnancy. Then there's the whole business of birth-one-upmanship. As Jane Garvey recently commented on Radio 4's *Woman's Hour*, we wouldn't expect a man to undergo a hernia operation without anaesthetic. Nor would we extract an infected appendix or rotten tooth without anaesthetic – what would be the point? The miracle that is modern-day science has created methods of pain relief, epidurals, Caesareans – none of which make childbirth an enjoyable process, but they do exist. So why all the preaching about drug-free labour? Is it superior to undergo second-degree perineal tears, to be left incontinent or worse – is it somehow more motherly to give birth in agony?

Successful women, earth-mothers, beautiful fertility goddesses do it naturally. In 2011 the Australian supermodel Miranda Kerr gave birth to her son Orlando after a drug-free labour lasting 27 hours – he weighed 10 lb. She later admitted that she was 'crazy' to do it without an epidural. The Brazilian supermodel Gisele Bundchen told the world about the blissful birth of her son: at home, in the bath, with no pain relief.

In October 2000, the actress Kate Winslet lied about the birth of her daughter Mia, saying she was born 'naturally and without complications'. But four years later, when she gave birth naturally to her son Joe, she admitted that her daughter had actually been delivered by emergency Caesarean section.

Arguably it's none of our business how Kate Winslet's babies were born – but her explanation is interesting: 'I've gone to great pains to cover it up,' she told the US magazine *Gotham* in 2004. 'But Mia was an emergency C-section. I just said that I had a natural birth because I was so completely traumatised by the fact that I hadn't given birth. I felt like a complete failure... There's this thing amongst women that if you can handle childbirth you can handle anything. I had never handled childbirth and I felt like in some way I couldn't enter the "powerful women's club".'

Having given birth to her son, she said, 'It was an amazing feeling having Joe naturally. Fourteen hours with no drugs at all, but then I had to have an epidural because I was so tired. It was an incredible birth. It was really triumphant.'

Commenting at the time, Mary Newburn of the National Childbirth Trust, said: 'No woman should ever feel a failure and it's terribly sad to hear that. The fact is, if she ended up having an emergency Caesarean section, then something wasn't right with the labour. Women who don't give birth the way they would want to either blame themselves or think that others will see it as a stigma.'

Winslet's story shed light on the pressures that she, and many women, feel to have the perfect birth. Female friends of mine have spoken of their determination to have an entirely drug-free labour and delivery. When this doesn't go according to plan, as most labours don't, and they're howling for an epidural/Caesarean/gun, they castigate themselves. Despite the fact that they've gone through the most intense pain of their lives; despite the fact that they have produced a real live baby. 'I tried so hard,' a friend of mine told me, in tears, following her 23-hour labour, failed induction and emergency Caesarean. 'I wanted to do it right, but the baby just wouldn't turn. I feel like I've failed.'

Why on earth should anyone's pregnancy make them feel guilty; how did needing a medical procedure become an admission of failure? Where pregnancy used to be a private matter between an expectant mother and her doctor, it's now become another one of the achievement-markers by which we judge women. I *do* think women should feel proud of giving birth. But I *don't* think they should feel ashamed of not doing it 'properly'.

Maybe we should all start saying *none of your business* when colleagues, friends or mothers-in-law ask about our childbirths. As the Vagenda feminists are fond of saying: STAY OUT OF OUR VAGINAS.

*

Not content with their triumphant births and near instantaneous baby-weight-loss, the final blow is how unmarked these successful women's bodies are by pregnancy. Their nine-month gestations seem to leave no trace. The supermodel-mother Miranda Kerr was back on the catwalk weeks after giving birth, modelling Victoria's Secret underwear.

Other celebrity mothers are snapped looking bikini-taut on the beach, and their stomachs simply do not look saggy, battered, or even stretched. Their hips do not widen with birth, their abdominal muscles do not develop an overhang, their Caesarean scar does not pucker or grow whiskery hairs (as a friend of mine reports hers has done). Apparently their breasts do not leak, and their belly buttons do not pop out. The livid stretch marks are nowhere to be seen. Rationally, we know these rich, successful women have a lot of help with their newborns and their post-natal bodies. They have personal trainers, chefs, nutritionists, nannies, housekeepers, personal assistants – possibly the odd nip-and-tuck after the birth – but that doesn't help. Perhaps we need to take a step back and realise that we don't need to aspire to those kinds of standards of perfection; perhaps we need to rejoice in the fact that we're free to be less than perfect.

It was headline news recently when the actress Kate Hudson admitted that she struggled to lose weight after her first pregnancy. This time, reports the *Daily Mail*, 'she put in the hard work, and it has most certainly paid off'. The star divulged: 'I devoted six hours a day to a vigorous workout regime. I would do 45 or 55 minutes of cardio then an hour of Pilates or yoga, three times a day.'

Um. OK. Most new mothers have barely six minutes a day to themselves, let alone six hours for a vigorous workout regime. Let alone the energy.

*

Of course there are more pressing issues in the world than a bunch of pampered celebrities who are obsessed with losing weight.

Their bodies are their careers and they have to look amazing – so what does it matter to the rest of us? We have real lives to live, relationships and families, children to bring up, jobs to hold down. And yet it *does* matter, because it filters down to the rest of us, with the powerful message that achievement is correlated to physical perfection. The beauty premium is an inescapable fact. Successful women are beautiful, groomed, and, above all, thin. So where does this message come from, and who can we blame? The reality is that we get the media we deserve – in others words, we vote with our wallets. Similarly, we get the celebrity culture and the magazines and the television we want. It is disingenuous and illogical to blame the modern media for their sexist attitudes to women: they are simply giving us, the readers, what we ask for. Presumably if we didn't want it, we wouldn't buy it.

Of course it's not that simple: culture and public opinion are a two-way street; we are influenced by, as well as influencers of, the media we consume. The power of advertising cannot be ignored; this is a multi-billion-dollar industry whose purpose is to sell us stuff. Young girls and teenagers are particularly vulnerable to celebrity endorsement, product placement and unrealistic media images.

But what about our own thoughts about ourselves and other women? If we're ever to find role models to whom we can relate, we need to call a halt to the constant building-up and pulling-down of women in the public eye. We need to recognise those emotions of jealousy and *Schadenfreude*. We need somehow to block the thought: *she's looking fat*. We need to stop enjoying the stories about break-ups, or failure, or weight gain. We need to stop making other women's lives harder. And if we're ever to reach a healthier relationship with our own bodies and weight, we need to look at what we define as beauty, and happiness, and success.

CONCLUSION

If I'm not thinking about my weight or calories, I'm either sleeping or dead. As long as I'm getting thinner, I'm cool.

This was two teenagers I recently overheard on a London bus. It's an alarming statement: sad, funny and ridiculous all at the same time, and perhaps truer for many of us than we'd care to admit. Because losing weight is a goal which unites the majority of women and men. Most people would like to be thinner.

But why? What does thin represent, and why is it so important to us? When you look at all the diets and advertisements and celebrity magazines, the yo-yo struggles and body-hatred and unhappiness, we have to ask, what are we really looking for here? Back to that conundrum: if losing weight is the answer, what is the question?

All the education, liberation and confidence in the world cannot seem to free us from the belief that thinner is somehow better. From weight to age, fashion to beauty, surgery to exercise, we've seen what all these dictatorships are doing to women: the imperatives to diet constantly, to consume only the most expensive organic food, to purify and detox on a regular basis, to exercise furiously, to find and marry the perfect man,

CONCLUSION

and then effortlessly produce babies, to be confident without
being strident, to be professionally ambitious and successful
without being pushy or unfeminine, to be naturally beautiful,
impeccably dressed and made-up, to stay young despite the
fact that we all get older, to conceal grey hairs, wrinkles and
any other signs of ageing, by surgical means if necessary... and
above all, to be thin.

Put like that, the situation for women seems fairly dire. Looking
back at the arguments of writers such as Simone de Beauvoir in
the 1940s and 1950s, Betty Friedan in the 1960s, Germaine Greer
in the 1970s and 1980s, Naomi Wolf in the 1990s – so much of
what they demanded, in terms of women's liberation at work and
at home, has been achieved. And what has that left?

It has left a paradox. Having broken down so many barriers,
we've created others to fill the void. We have fought for our
independence, we've struggled to control our own lives, our
careers, property and finances, but at the same time we have
introduced a way of holding ourselves back: a profound lack
of physical confidence. How perverse and self-sabotaging this
anxiety over our appearance is: at a time when we're materially
freer than ever before, we have a whole new set of rules to make
ourselves unhappy: hunger, perfection, thinness.

And yet, there is cause for optimism. Across the world, a new
wave of feminism is taking hold: irreverent, feisty, and fuelled
by social media. The Vagenda (vagendamag.blogspot.co.uk) is
a feminist blog which satirises the portrayal of women in the
media, and women's magazines in particular. Everyday Sexism
(www.everydaysexism.com) is a website which compiles accounts
of the casual discrimination and harassment women face on a
day-to-day basis – not rape or abuse, just stories of sexism
faced by ordinary women in ordinary places. No More Page 3
(nomorepage3.org) is a campaign demanding that *The Sun* 'drop

the bare boobs' in Rupert Murdoch's bestselling tabloid. The woman who launched the campaign, Lucy Holmes, asked a group of men for their reactions to *The Sun*'s Page 3. One said, 'I feel like a perv, I turn the page.' Another laughed and said, 'Look at the tits on that.' It is this dehumanising of women into a body with a pair of 'tits' that encourages men to see women, and some women to see themselves, as sex objects.

There may be cause for optimism in fashion too, with a major department store chain deciding to employ models who don't fit the conventionally perfect mould. Debenhams is taking a stand against 'size zero tyranny' by using plus-size, petite and older models, and even women with disabilities, to promote their fashion ranges. The store said it wants to help shoppers feel better about their bodies by boycotting unrealistic 'waif culture' images. Whether this signals a genuine milestone towards wider representations of beauty, only time will tell... but it's a step in the right direction.

*

We have more freedom and choice than ever before, yet ever more is expected of us. Male and female roles are changing, and the way we relate to each other is subtly changing too. Men are not redundant – of course not – but there's no doubt that women are less dependent on men for their financial and social security. If you decide to go it alone as a single woman, or if you haven't found the right relationship, these days you are not a social outcast, destitute or condemned to a life in your parents' attic. As gender dynamics have shifted, it does create other complications, and women are starting to reassess their own role in society, with family and with themselves, their aspirations and ambitions, their bodies and their identities.

It can be hard to find a middle way. It's like the old saying goes: everything in moderation.

And yet, moderation is hard, when we are surrounded by abundance. Simply being a woman in the twenty-first century is a balancing act – being feminine but also being strong – giving and receiving pleasure – caring for others while respecting yourself – protecting yourself from violation and exploitation – sending out the right or wrong 'signals' – eating healthily but not too heartily – being successful but not too pushy – being aware of others but secure in yourself – loving without being dependent – female without being vulnerable... it's complicated.

It was a century ago that Virginia Woolf asked, 'Why are women... so much more interesting to men than men are to women?' This isn't necessarily fair on men – lots of them are interesting too – but there is something wonderful, and highly perceptive and sensitive and generous about women. I recently took part in a Channel 4 Roundtable Discussion on feminism and body image with a group of female journalists, MPs and policy makers, and came away feeling absolutely inspired. This is often the case when you gather a group of women together: the results can be amazing.

And yet, frustrating as it is to admit, women make life difficult for other women. Much of the despair is self-inflicted – the desire to be superslim comes from other women or magazines or ourselves, not from men. When we're united we could move mountains; when we're divided, and bitching, and jealous, we destroy each other's self-esteem.

Women are intensely contradictory: this is part of what makes being a woman so interesting and so impossible. We rail against trashy celebrity culture, we complain about the media's relentless bitch-fest, and their glorification of unhealthy, unrealistic size-zero models, and yet we write, purchase and avidly consume precisely the body-fodder pumped out by these magazines. We're opinionated, educated and sceptical: we know about the airbrushing, we can see through the advertising, and yet we continue to cough up for anti-ageing snake oil in French packaging. We say we want to see 'real' women with 'fuller' figures, yet secretly we'd do anything to be one of the perfect ones. We watch semi-naked pop stars booty-dancing while singing about being 'Independent Women'; we kid ourselves this is girl power.

We say that age doesn't matter, that beauty comes from within, and yet we're full of anxiety about ageing, and horribly critical of our own bodies. We pay men in white coats to fix us up on the operating table – yes, we pay thousands of pounds for the privilege of unnecessary surgery. Rationally we understand that most diets fail, and that eating disorders are hell – and yet we're constantly trying to lose weight.

This is strangest of all: we know that being skinny won't automatically make our lives perfect (no, it won't) and yet we tell ourselves it will. We bleat about self-acceptance while choosing this pointless cycle of guilt about food, eating and appetites. Many of us live in daily hatred of our own bodies, ruled by the number on the scales and the reflection in the mirror.

So this isn't a manifesto for women's liberation, as such. Fifty years since Betty Friedan wrote *The Feminine Mystique*, 'feminism' is still perceived by many as a dirty word. A recent survey, conducted by Christina Scharff at the University of London, found that the term 'feminism' 'provokes unease and even hostility'. A 2012 survey by Netmums found that only one in seven women identify themselves as 'feminists' (with younger women least likely to). And these are only the latest in a long line of studies which show that the F-word is widely unpopular. Many women feel the term is old-fashioned or irrelevant, and they can't imagine a time when men and women weren't equal. Others view the ideology of feminism as aggressive, divisive, and even oppressive towards men. It seems that we like the results of feminism – personal freedom and relative equality – but feel uncomfortable with the label itself.

*

Remember that saying: 'Never ask the advice of someone who has not had your kind of trouble'? When it comes to recovery from eating disorders, I try to steer clear of offering advice. I don't have the secret, and it can be hard enough keeping myself on track, let alone others. But recently, after several frantic emails from a reader (detailing her entire weight history, from a high of 14 stone to a low of 6 stone, and a current weight of 9 stone), I broke my own rules on giving advice. In case you're going through the same thing, here's what I said:

> *Throw out your scales. I know you'll think that's dangerous/ risky/mad, and your weight will spin out of control, but I promise you it won't. You say you're stuck around 9 stone – surely your body is telling you that you have a happy, healthy weight. You tell me you're about to marry the man you love; why not stop torturing yourself with all this leaping on and off the scales, and let yourself live?*
>
> *And who actually cares whether you're 8 stone or 9 stone? You do, and it's making you miserable, but no-one else can even see it: your weight is NOT printed on your forehead each morning. You say you weigh yourself compulsively, that you 'have to know'... Maybe it's time to look at the control issue, rather than trying to maintain an impossibly low weight. Honestly, think about it. Your scales are the problem, not your size.*

Of course I knew she wouldn't follow my advice. Her response came back, typically anorexic – and I mean that fondly, because I recognise it. With permission, here's her reply:

My immediate reaction to 'throw out your scales': that's too scary. Risky. My worst fear is going back to being as big as I was. And anyway, you have never been fat. Before I started this (initially sensible!) diet, I was a size 18. My problem is that I cannot judge my own size – in the mirror, I see someone huge. But I see your point entirely. Why should my day and my mood be dictated by what those numbers tell me every time I strip off and stand on that cold glass surface? I reason with your logic... until the fear comes back. What if I lose control? I know that food should be enjoyable, but what if I just keep gaining weight? In some aspects, I do want to recover, and in others, I don't. The risk is too high. Imagine having to buy bigger clothes. It's all such a slippery slope.

Like every anorexic, she has this illusion that she's in control. But she's not. Her bathroom scales are. It's her struggle, and I wish her all the strength she needs to win through – I know how hard it is.

I get so many emails like this, from women and men who are dreadfully unhappy about their weight. There's probably not much point in telling others what to do, but what I always want to say to these strangers with anorexia, bulimia and worse, but in a more eloquent form, is: stop right now... just give it up and don't waste the years ahead, and don't kid yourself that there's some point to being hungry or that it gives you any control over things because it doesn't and life is uncontrollable and eating disorders are just another way of hiding.

Like many women, I have spent too long worrying about things like eating and weight. When I look back, I'm not even sure why. It was never about the actual shape of my body; rather a disrespectful attitude to what I needed: food, rest, care. The simple things that every person needs. I developed a seriously messed-up relationship with my appetite, deciding that if I was hungry I must be weak, and if I ate, I was giving in. A completely pointless battle with myself. It sounds insignificant, but throwing away my bathroom scales was as crucial to my recovery as starting to eat again. I abandoned the morning weigh-in, and in doing so I freed myself from the daily dose of guilt. One small step for me, one giant leap for recovery.

*

The question is not what woman can achieve; the question is what we *allow ourselves* to achieve. There can be no doubt that women are as intelligent, ambitious and talented as men (if not more so). So how do we end the self-hatred and the sniping; how can we be more collaborative – more, dare I say it, sisterly?

One of the simplest strategies to remember is that another woman's achievements do not diminish you in any way. Unless you're in direct competition for a job, a gold medal, or an award, their success does not mean your failure. This sounds obvious but it's fundamental to the way we think, and the way that collectively we're so often our worst enemies. I was recently talking to a friend who is trying for a baby. 'I had this revelation,' she said, 'it's not a competition. Every time someone else got pregnant I'd feel depressed, until one day it dawned on me: there isn't a finite amount of baby dust. It was a breakthrough – realising that them getting pregnant doesn't in any way prevent me from getting pregnant too.'

And it's the same with achievement: there isn't a finite amount of female success. Someone else doing well should not make us feel threatened or inadequate. On the contrary, the more that women excel, the more glass ceilings we can all smash through, collectively. It's a cliché, but we are stronger when we're together. It's too easy to turn our own insecurities outwards, to criticise other women for trying too hard, or letting themselves go, or being too fat or too thin... but in the end, we feel worse, not better, about ourselves. Most of life is hard – we're all engaged in putting a brave face on our anxieties, most days. But if we open up a little, and trust and support each other, we will find that there is strength in numbers.

*

As we've seen, the tentacles of the Ministry of Thin – and Diets, Detox and the rest – reach far into our lives. From childhood we absorb messages about weight and appearance, and they're almost impossible to eradicate. Even if we could ban all magazine, film, TV and Internet images, we cannot undo the cultural pressures to look a certain way. There is an overwhelming consensus on what 'attractive' looks like: slim, symmetrical, smooth. Is it any wonder that we have internalised the message that sagging, or having lines, or going grey is somehow shameful, when there are so many ways to 'conceal' or 'reverse' the visible signs of ageing? 'Fat' and 'old' are no longer statements of fact, but admissions of failure. For many, even eating a hearty meal is a guilt-ridden act.

Look at what the Ministry of Thin can do. It can cause us to hate ourselves, to starve or spend hours in the gym, even undergo risky surgery. It can make us feel inadequate and unattractive, telling us we are failures, and ugly, and weak. It sets us against ourselves, profoundly at war with our own bodies. It imprisons us in a lifelong cycle of weight loss and gain; a war we'll never win, and which will never make us happy.

Of course there are still women and men with the confidence to accept themselves as they are – and that's fantastic – but we face an increasingly narrow standard of what is physically acceptable. Simply liking yourself has become controversial. The growth of disordered eating, depression, self-harm and body dysmorphia is a reminder that women and men of all ages are struggling to reconcile their bodies and minds. Ask yourself, honestly, if you could choose, how would you look? You would probably choose thinner over fatter, and younger over older…

Of all the pressures we face, being thin is probably the hardest to ignore. Even if we ignore the media images and the miracle diets, we still have that inner voice reminding us that thinner is better. You know that carping voice: *if only you ate less, you greedy pig, if only you worked out harder, you lazy cow, if only, if only, you'd be slimmer, fitter, less flabby, more desirable…* But really, the most desirable thing is being happy in our skin. That inner voice is a bully, and a coward, and it won't fade easily. Sometimes all we can do is put our fingers in our ears and shout: *lalala, shut up, not listening; I'm eating the cake because I want to.*

I know that a state of absolute self-acceptance is well-nigh impossible: even the greatest 'beauty' has hang-ups, and it's much harder for the rest of us to love our flaws. Perhaps all we can do is to appreciate our bodies, and to avoid the damaging language of self-hate; to look beyond the superficial and stop judging, measuring, weighing up. Youth, with its firm skin and smooth lines, is enjoyable of course, but it doesn't last forever. Above all, let's remember what matters: friendship, family, love; and what doesn't matter quite so much: perfect nails, skin, or hair, being size zero or cellulite-free.

The Ministry of Thin is a trap, a horribly powerful force in our lives, inside our heads. And crucially, anyone can be caught in this trap: fat or curvy or slim or skeletal, no one is immune.

The endless battle with our weight and appetite is deeply self-destructive, and we need to call a halt. We need to start valuing our bodies for what they do and think and feel, rather than how they look, how they compare to others, and how they fall short. We'll never completely erase those external beauty standards of course, but we can decide to ignore the internal monologue of body-hatred.

I know it's not easy. Until more recently than I care to admit, deep-down I needed to be thin. Not for the sake of thinness itself, but because I somehow felt apologetic about being hungry and needing food; about taking up space in the world.

So, you may well be thinking, what does a woman who suffered from anorexia for ten years have to tell me about self-acceptance? How can she call herself a feminist if she spent all that time trying to stay thin? I'm conscious of the contradictions: I know only too well how the Ministry of Thin has affected my own life. But I live in the same world as you, I'm as self-aware as you are, and I know that my experience is not uncommon these days.

Getting very thin made me very unhappy; I am still picking up the pieces. But it taught me about resilience, and how to live inside my own body. People often talked to me about 'willpower', as if having anorexia was somehow strong. This is wrong. It is standing up to the Ministry of Thin which takes real strength.

Of course it's not simple. It takes a thick skin not to feel inadequate in these image-obsessed times, but I believe we face a fundamental choice. Either we can continue in this state of perpetual discomfort, or we can change the way we think and talk, and gradually, the way we feel about our bodies. It is time for us to put the Ministry of Thin, and all the other ministries of self-doubt and fear, out of business, once and for all. Time to find something more absorbing and rewarding – and for god's sake, more interesting – than the pursuit of thin.

CONCLUSION

Remember the saying: *treat others as you would be treated*? Well how about this: *treat yourself as you would treat others*. A little kindness and respect for our own bodies could go a long way. We are, all of us, worth care and nurture and food. The strongest thing I have ever done is not to lose weight, but to gain it back again. It has taken me a long time to look myself in the eye and say: *you matter*. But I do. And so do you.

RESOURCES

10 Steps to Positive Body Image from the National Eating Disorders Association (USA)
www.nationaleatingdisorders.org/10-steps-positive-body-image

Age UK
www.ageuk.org.uk

Anorexia & Bulimia Care
www.anorexiabulimiacare.org.uk

Beat
www.b-eat.co.uk
Beat is the leading organization in the UK providing information and help on all aspects of eating disorders, including anorexia, bulimia, binge-eating and related conditions. Message boards and useful resources for sufferers, families and carers.

BBC Health pages
www.bbc.co.uk/health

Depression Alliance
www.depressionalliance.org

Everyday Sexism
www.everydaysexism.com

Men Get Eating Disorders Too
www.mengetedstoo.co.uk
A national charity dedicated to representing and supporting the needs of men with eating disorders. Excellent source of information and advice for boys and men of all ages, with friendly message boards and peer support.

Mental Health Foundation
www.mentalhealth.org.uk

Mind
www.mind.org.uk

National Centre for Eating Disorders
www.eating-disorders.org.uk
Provides information and professional training in the treatment of anorexia, bulimia, binge and compulsive overeating, orthorexia and obesity.

NHS Choices
www.nhs.uk/Conditions/Eating-disorders/
www.nhs.uk/Livewell/mentalhealth/

No More Page 3
nomorepage3.org

Samaritans
www.samaritans.org

SANE
www.sane.org.uk

Something Fishy
www.something-fishy.org
Popular pro-recovery support website with community boards and frequently asked questions. Information on eating disorders and mental health; definitions, signs and symptoms, physical dangers.

The Vagenda
vagendamag.blogspot.co.uk

ACKNOWLEDGEMENTS

Many people have provided support during the writing of this book. Particular thanks are due to the following:

To all at Summersdale Publishers, especially Alastair, Claire, Lizzie, Suzanne and Debbie, and to Stephen Wildish for the cover design. Special thanks to Abbie Headon and Jennifer Barclay for their editorial insight and friendship.

Thanks to some marvellous individuals: Nick Breakell, Darren Bird, Libby Courtice, Rita Guenigault, Susan Archer, Beth Wilson, Mickie Rose, Lucy Fry, Ceara Hayden, Nicky Rodway, Raelene Sheppard, Valerie Janitch, Tamsin Hickson and Bunny Schendler.

Thanks to the self-styled Apples: Miranda, Meg, Thinky and Sara, fruity and brilliant to the core. And thanks to all my Twitter friends: far too many to mention, and far too many hours tweeting when I should be writing. It's impossible now that the British Library has Wi-Fi.

To TGW, and Marie Schendler, in loving memory.

Thank you to my sisters, Katie and Alice, and my brothers, Philip and Trim. You're the best.

Finally, to my parents Cecil and Jean Woolf. There for me, through thick and thin.

Have you enjoyed this book?
If so, why not write a review on your favourite website?

If you're interested in finding out more about our books, find us
on Facebook at **Summersdale Publishers** and
follow us on Twitter at **@Summersdale**.

Thanks very much for buying this Summersdale book.

www.summersdale.com